Beyond Epigenetics

Introduction:

First, a warning: If you expect to get anything like the full intent of this (and my other books), you must watch the referenced videos. This is a fully interactive book and I keep it short with no bibliography for good reason,

Welcome to this new book, Beyond Epigenetics, the third in this series that incorporates the most profound advancement in healing known to man, maybe ever, certainly in modern history.

Herein, we discuss the perceived new fractally-based quantum science as taught by Dan Nelson, combined with my friend, Rich Prices's spiritual ability to rise beyond the subconscious level and diagnose illness from the high planes of what some term as God-Consciousness.

Background:

The first two books were not totally original ideas in our search for health. Still, the HL MSM, as introduced, was virtually unknown to nearly everyone and certainly was unknown to even the most informed alternative professional. However, the horse farmer who introduced it to me has proven to have been thoroughly on top of his game and as new facts are revealed with new studies, his wisdom was indeed far reaching, original in its detail, and always up until now, has proven itself as accurate.

The first book, "It's the Liver Stupid" explained and introduced the now well established HL MSM protocol. It is further expanded upon herein with some new work, studies, and commentary. It also focused on Undenatured Whey Protein Isolates, and the Low Carb Diet protocols along with many adjutants.

The second book, "Methylation, Awareness, and You" explained the cutting edge methylation sequences and epigenetics and revealed the mechanisms behind, especially, the HL MSM Protocol of the first book.

Rich first learned about quantum healing after attending a conference in Niagra Falls in 2013 after this author encouraged him to do so. Dan Nelson was probably the foremost quantum scientist on earth in terms of what he had accomplished at the time in using the technology. However, the work that Rich is doing now, no doubt now surpasses Dan's. He uses the same CP4U-F (Crystal Pack 4 Unit Fractal) with different proprietary programs, and sometimes two, in order to contain the information required to heal and we use four for the car program.

Herein, we discuss the perceived new, fractally-based quantum science as taught by Dan Nelson combined with Rich's intuitive ability.

This book, "Beyond Epigentics" then discusses an original, fractally-based method of diagnosis that my friend, Richard S. Price devised. Using this, he combines a fractal healing system that Rich, loosely based on the work of Dan Nelson and expands on it on way that no one else likely ever could.

With this, I submit that this new work takes healing to realms heretofore unattainable by conventional science and expands it. While Epigenetics is still very much cutting edge and best expressed by Dr. Bruce Lipton, the work herein has never been documented prior to this book. Furthermore, while it is new, it has been applied to many people with such parasitic diseases as Lymes and Malaria and their related infections and has successfully resolved them in just a matter of hours.

Not only has Rich applied the above technology to help people be cured of these and other devastating diseases, we together have used it as a machine enhancement device that improves car performance. Thus, in a sense, it "cures" engine ills also. These systems, we have come to realize, are very predictable and reliable. In every case, they cause our test VW Jetta TDI to record mileage figures never commonly seen, no matter what the driven the conditions are. So, no matter what the machine, a human body or a diesel engine, they work extraordinarily well.

Table of Contents

The Gene Code
http://en.wikipedia.org/wiki/Genetic_code

The genetic code is the set of rules by which information is encoded within genetic material, that is, DNA and mitochondrial RNA (mRNA) sequences are translated into proteins by living cells. Biological decoding is accomplished by ribosomes and these link amino acids in an order specified by mRNA, using transfer RNA (tRNA) molecules to carry them and to read the mRNA, three nucleotides at a time.

The important note here is that the genetic code is highly similar among all organisms and can be expressed in a simple table with 64 entries (per Wikipedia). Furthermore, this code, as applied to the human genome, is far more simple than previously anticipated prior to gene sequencing. In fact, in sequencing the code, it was discovered that the human genome was no more complex than that of much more simple animals. Furthermore, in some cases, our code is less complex than even some worms, to the surprise of virtually all scientists involved prior to the sequencing. That is, the anticipation was that it would be many times that of any other biology on earth. The implication herein, then, is that it is "quantum events," or epigenetics, actually guide our complexity far more than genes. Thus, we are in control of our own demise in ways that were never before anticipated.

Furthermore, prior to sequencing, the great hope in decoding the sequences was that this would eventually result in curing all disease, especially autoimmune diseases and cancer. This, of course, never occurred, but as the below publication predicts, today's science still grasps this "great hope" tightly even though it cannot ever occur. So we see that science today has become more of a wish than a fact as we waste billions of dollars on hopes that have no promise as Dr. Bruce Lipton points out in his talks so cleverly.

In the field of cancer, the greatest hope here, very little has changed following the sequencing. The "new" chemo treatments, now called "targeted gene therapies," **http://www.cancer.gov/cancertopics/treatment/types/targeted-therapies/targeted-therapies-fact-sheet**, are still basically poisons to the human body just as the first chemo treatment, "mustard gas" of WWI was years ago. To quote the above link: *"Scientists had expected that targeted cancer therapies would be less toxic than traditional chemotherapy drugs because cancer cells are more dependent on the targets than are normal cells. However, targeted cancer therapies can have substantial side effects."* The point here is that they all still do have these side effects, just as their own literature points out, and they are life threatening when taken as a protocol.

Should you disagree with the above, read the "side effects" of these individual chemodrugs, as published by each of their pharmaceutical manufacturers. The fact remains that these cancer drugs are the same killers that they always were to some degree. So the bottom line is: While all chemodrugs will initially, and often (but not always), as mustard gas did years ago, cause tumors to temporarily recede, eventually, when taken long-term, as virtually all of these drug companies report of their own drugs, they can (and generally do), cause death. So at this point, the idea that genetics makes them more safe has now generally become a marketing ploy and not the established fact that they want you to believe. Moreover, these, so called, targeted drugs are among the most expensive drugs in the world and anything to help sell them will be touted by their owners. So, no, this is not the scientific advancement that the public has been led to believe. This is just an anticipated scientific advancement that never panned out. It is an idea and hope that was generally anticipated by the scientific world that never happened.

Genetics in Medicine (GIM)

http://www.nature.com/gim/index.html
Genetics in Medicine (GIM) is the official journal of the American College of Medical Genetics and Genomics. This monthly journal teaches a genetic medicine,

including topics on chromosome abnormalities, metabolic diseases, single gene disorders, genetic susceptibility to common complex diseases, etc.

When the gene code was broken as described above, this was the great hope. This and similar publications still teach that something will come out of this. However, despite the setback, what has actually appeared is quite useful and as follows, yet none of this was anticipated by the above work (almost in opposition to the their setback):

Epigentics and Methylation Therapies

One of the huge strides that arose from this gene sequencing was in our understanding that we, as individuals, can actually change sections (known as SNIPS) of the gene code on a subconscious level. Thus, the idea that the code was determined and everything was set, was and is incorrect and changing it is within our abilities to correct. These methylation sequences are affected by various supplements, foods, and especially, our conscious minds. But they are changed only on the unconscious level. Thus, the popular concept that one can will themselves well is equally incorrect. No one makes subconscious changes intentionally, but we can set up the conditions to make them occur.

Beyond Epigenetics

The above introduction explains how Rich Price, introduced above, can rise above the subconscious mind and make actual changes to it so as to effect mental and physical health in ways previously not understood by science. While this ability can be taught to select few, it is not likely to be within the knowledge of most health care practitioners today. However, the goal, herein, is to help change this.

Dietary Oils... The Good and the Bad

The important aspect of the story below is that it demonstrates just how controlling the commercialized side of health and especially the food and drug industry is and has been historically. Margarine, our target topic here, was first introduced more than one hundred years ago and the idea that cholesterol was a heart health problem arose with the acceptance of this food. In fact, it still manages to be sold as a healthy food substitute for butter despite the obvious deception used in selling the product:
Margarine is quite simply, whipped-up cottonseed oil, and cottonseed oil is: Wouldn't you know it, an unregulated waste by-product of cotton production? There is probably nothing inherent in margarine that could even remotely be considered healthy or even considered as food, yet it is still being sold today and touted as a heart healthy butter substitute.

10

Below is the authors edited version of this margarine story that is repeated many times on the web in different versions:

The dairy industry was extremely powerful in the 1900's. Thus, this industry controlled and affected dairy and marketing practices with an iron hand.
http://en.wikipedia.org/wiki/Cottonseed_oil

The cotton raisers had this cottonseed oil by-product that they were unable to even dump in the ground. It was an ugly gray material that had no resemblance to butter. However, someone got the idea that they could whip it up and sell it as a butter substitute... As a way to get rid of the mess and even earn profits in the process.

So they came out with new less objectionable appearing products and, along the way, found a PhD scientist whom they managed to get on the cover of Life Magazine who offered it up as a cure for heart disease. His age-old theory derived from a rabbit study later was accepted by the AMA as the "Cholesterol Theory."

You can read about the man, Ancel Keys and his now infamous theory here:
http://junkscience.com/2013/05/09/putting-a-stake-through-the-cholesterol-theory-of-heart-disease/

So margarine was pushed onto the public as one of the great ways to beat heart disease. Along the way, all unsaturated fats took this position alongside Margarine as well. So corn oil became known as a heart-healthy oil. No one at the time even paid attention to the transfats that they become at high temperatures when they were used as cooking oils.

Digressing, the butter industry would allow no part of this and they came back with a vengeance. Their first move was to disallow the cotton seed people from coloring their ugly mess with yellow food dyes to make it look like butter.
So the answer from the cottonseed people was in their providing a coloring "kit." This kit included a packet of this yellow food dye that the housewife mixed in with the cotton seed oil after buying it.

Later, of course, after they managed to convince the entire medical industry (with the advice of Keys) that Cholesterol is a killer. Thus, they proceeded to sell their margarine colored yellow and even came out with such clever ads as. "I can't believe it's not butter" as they continued their charade to push it as heart-healthy.

However, please believe them: It is "not butter" and it will eventually help kill you if you keep using it. In fact, Cholesterol, as discussed herein in several places and touted by the wonderful Dr. Stephanie Seneff, is a major part of your brain (Alzheimer's anyone?) and, as she points out in her many You Tube videos: Cholesterol is an incredibly essential part of your diet. If it is lacking, you will become diseased. Your mind will deteriorate, your circulatory system will harden, and your heart will fail from overwork, just as she and others predict.

Listen to Dr. Stephanie Seneff's interview
https://www.youtube.com/watch?v=I-jJn-4jUxg
Above, she discusses the need for higher cholesterol (and as much as you can get). In fact, including more cholesterol in your diet, as she discusses, will result in the lowering of heart disease rates and lower blood pressures. Of course, this is just the opposite of what we are taught, but this will eventually become a very well established fact as we move forward.

We are not herbivores. Look at your teeth, please. Meat is a very dense brain food. We need the good fats and those are cholesterols in our diets (yes, these are the saturated fats shunned for so many years by the mainstream). Getting them back into your diet will help add years to your life as long as it comes from healthy sources (wherein lies the rub).

But herein lies the key today, good sources of fats are harder to find than in the '50's. Now that feed lots have become more common and drugs are necessarily employed in the beef producing processes just to keep the cattle alive. Note that cats and dogs will fight to get those saturated animal fats that you throw out as you pass up the fats and eat the lean meat. Are they more intelligent than you?

The best saturated fat, however, may just be coconut oil and it seems to make many things taste better when used in cooking. Additionally, it is very resistant to high heat. Thus, unlike the vegetable oils, it does not become a transfat easily. Therefore, it is often recommended by many healthcare professionals in the know, even though many medschools and dieticians still teach dangerous dietary information today after a half century of bad advice.

Today, the AMA today, generally, still backs this cottonseed industry (along with Statins, of course, the most successful drug on the market):
http://www.cottonseedoiltour.com/facts/
http://www.cottonseed.com/publications/facts.asp

A longer and more involved historical version of the above story is available at:
http://mentalfloss.com/article/25638/surprisingly-interesting-history-margarine

Below, Dr. Mercola's dialog agrees with the above commentary:
http://articles.mercola.com/herbal-oils/cottonseed-oil.aspx

Cancer Theory

The below and above story are introduced early herein in hopes that the eyes of the doubters will be opened. That is, they will read the references and thus will begin to understand the facts. These all carry billion dollar price tags, so they will remain very slow to be uncovered, but this is the reality and the truth is coming out. The transfat story was the first bolt from the mainstream teaching. More will follow.

Cancer and Fats

Now realize that cancer, to begin with, is a multifaceted disease.

Today, this so-called disease, cancer, is seen as rapidly increasing and uncontrolled cell division with no real known cause other than bad genes and, maybe, too many toxins. So, no one today has a clue as to why cancer ever occurs, for the most part. Seldom does anyone even offer a suggestion as to why. Instead, all you hear is that it is a very complex disease that stems mostly from genes, even

15

though billions of dollars have been spent in studying it (and certainly more than on any other disease).

Below, I offer the cause, as I look at it in a very different light, based on the contention that our bodies are actually quantum machines that generally heal themselves if given the opportunity. Agreed, this theory is a radical departure from mainstream descriptions, but it does begin to make sense compared to the others (who throw up their hands), when you analyze it:

Cancer is a naturally occurring reaction to toxic chemical build-ups. Furthermore, do to the fact that it lowers immune response, it is always accompanied by invasive nanobacteria, fungal, viral infections, and parasites. When these co-infections are removed, it gives the body a far better chance of overcoming the toxins that initially caused the problem. In fact, as Royal Rife proved in the 1940's: In most cases, the people relieved of these opportunistic invaders survive and the cancer disappears.

However, I submit that the cancer will generally dissipate if either the invaders or the toxins are removed as long as the diet is sufficient to provide the dietary sulfur and fats needed for overall wellness. Therefore, in every case, if a person is relieved of one or both conditions and it has the

16

required nutrients, there will be no more, so called "disease."

The problem here is (and always it has been true since ancient Greek times), that cancer has been considered a biological and, more recently, genetic mistake. However, this theory holds that cancer is just another system of biological survival. The bottom line then, is that cancer is a condition in which the body is attempting to relieve itself of toxins from an overloaded liver. In this process, these host invaders infect the body as secondary infections (that in the 1940's, Rife interpreted as primary, in his work).

Below are some rather well established generalities pointed out to back up the above proposed theory:

1. There is no such thing as cancer of the heart. Why? In its infinite wisdom, the body knows that the heart is essential, so it protects it at all cost.

2. Skin cancer occurs more often than any other. Why? The skin is the least important organ and the body can survive the longest when it is compromised. Certainly, any trauma can help contribute to toxic load and an invasion. However, the sun, when not overdone, now has been shown to have a proven anti-cancer effect.

3. Liver cancer is rare. Why? The liver is, by far, the most important organ in the order of survival in the human body as long as the heart keeps pumping. As the above theory states, the entire point behind cancer is an effort to assist in relieving the liver of toxins. The last resort then, by this definition, is liver cancer.

By extension: If you have liver cancer, then you are basically on the final track to death from toxic overload. Therefore, cancer is progressively most deadly according to the biological importance of the associated organ as determined by our super intelligent quantum bodies.

Continuing with the above, the human body is infinitely more intelligent than its conscious mind (or any doctor's mind). All sub-conscious intelligence, which, as mentioned, you can't readily affect, is higher knowledge and commonly inaccessible to the reactive lower mind. This is the basis of epigenetics, the newest, yet oldest and most profound of accepted science today. So quantum healing as discussed herein, along with the idea of epigentics, is the next step beyond epigenetics. Hang onto your hat as we begin the venture into the next step.

Curing Cancer Historically, The Quacks

Why cancer is not cured by doctors and how you might cure it using some historic as well as some more recent food and supplement methods:

https://www.youtube.com/watch?v=NAMYAoiCSsI

The Ojibwa tribe in the above video was probably still working with Quantum Science to some degree in their day. Thus they were still epigeneticists at heart in their time.

Essiac tea is simply an herbal mix. Essiac does not contain HL MSM. However, we know that my friend, Paul in New Zealand, who is probably the only cured, diagnosed S-4 Mesothelioma Case alive today, used just HL MSM, as described later along with a clean and careful diet. However, herbs contain mineral, vitamins, and phytochemicals and these can all deliver the necessary nutrients when done correctly.

You also must first realize that, at the time, there was no reason to believe that HL MSM would cure Paul of lung cancer that was apparent. Once you study how MSM works and you understand the Methylation Pathways (which I did not at the time), you know why this protocol works.

Furthermore, Paul's cure also should give you some insight into how cancer works as it did me and the few ever given this level of insight. I suggest that the key here is with the Methyl groups, not the sulfur, that turned the tide. Still, as Dr. Seneff tells you, the sulfur and cholesterol will help. These, when enhanced, raise the

19

body harmonics to new levels and thus perform in much the same way as quantum healing as introduced in the previous discussion. The end result, while not identical, is to balance the system and raise its harmonic levels and allow the body the freedom to heal.

Realize also that Paul was first attempting natural cures and without this combination, no cure could have likely occurred. So, yes, add essiac tea or its herbal mix if you are diagnosed with cancer. As I report herein, by using quantum frequencies as previously discussed, an instantaneous cancer reversal is quite possible and even likely. What Paul did was to introduce dietary healing frequencies into his body and thus balance his disharmonics using the HL MSM protocol.

Paul's problem reportedly began when he breathed in asbestos from brake drums while working on cars as a mechanic over a long period. The MSM, as we now understand it, helped remove this cancer causing problem from his lungs as it helped restore his methylation sequences and thus raise his harmonics. While this is a slower process, just as with Rich's methods, it is not just a treatment, it is also a long-term cure. That is, unless he were to reintroduce the offending asbestos back into his lungs, he is likely cured forever.

Some other well known cancer cures and treatments:

The Hoxey Story below is fun, but it's only a skin cancer cure. What I like about it is the Morris Fishbine part. Fishbine is that this is the very same guy who ran Royal Rife into bankruptcy. He was the head of the AMA and its spokesman in that time. Royal Rife, were he alive today, could do some of what my friend Rich Price does, but using extreme radio frequencies. These were lower level and heavy handed, but they were effective at killing some parasites. He attacked tumors directly and was able to accomplish his cancer cures (considered incurable by oncologists) 20 out of 22 cancer cases. Thus, he apparently killed offending secondary viruses, bacteria, and fungi and freed the patients of biological burden, thus curing their cancer.
https://www.youtube.com/watch?v=90rGPCXWHDk

Dr. Gerson was absolutely on point. He cured most diseases including cancer with just diet and was way ahead of his time. His book, "A Cancer Treatment," is awesome. The only concern here is with his only using a vegetarian diet, because a very low fat diet invites cancer and very few plants possess a full dietary complement. To this writer's view, Dr. Lawrence Fishbine should have been incarcerated for his actions. Gerson cured 50 out of 52 incurable cancer patients. The AMA hated this man. Most people are unlikely able to provide the dietary extremes that Gerson used and there are other measures that can help equally well or better.

21

http://www.amazon.com/Dr-Max-Gerson-Healing-Hopeless-ebook/dp/B002FB66DC

Laetrile may actually work, but will we ever know? One should not be too skeptical, given the real proof. This, could be explained by the "poison" factor that laetrile introduces, somewhat like mustard gas. Mistletoe (iscatore) injected would fall into the same category.
http://www.chrisbeatcancer.com/b17-laetrile-alternative-cancer-treatment-suppressed-50-years/

Shark cartilage may work also and the theory may prove out, but it is getting old in the teeth, thus the theory below holds more promise:

This is the lipo C idea as best as presented by Dr. Levy and it can't do a thing to harm like the above poisons might:
https://www.youtube.com/watch?v=z1kD3BolXnE

Next we have the most recent promise "baking soda," as promoted by Dr. Simoncini in Italy
My friend, Dr. Kevin Freeman and I actually talked directly with him on the phone. Unfortunately, he basically bailed out when he was put to the test. Obviously, cancer has its hangers on who move in when the body's immune system is down, so his argument may hold some water.

We decided that his basic ideas were not so far off, but still were limited. We know that chemo keeps cancer from ever going away totally, but has always retarded it for a time and that some sodium bicarbonate may be in order in getting rid of cancer. Last heard, Simoncini still practices, by the way, by hiring others who do his work.

So the above are the so called "quacks" who have been disregarded by mainstream medicine.
A common mainstream quote is: "We know how cancers behave? (Dr. Barrett, Quackwatch)
So we must ask, "If that is true, why the dismal record? Dr. Barrett, is a non-practicing psychologist making a living off of big pharma (who is paying him to offend people like Mercola). Quackwatch (his website) labels Mercola and the others above as quacks. This label is becoming a badge of honor in the attempt to bring good health. Unlike Mercola, Barrett does not apparently even practice medicine and has been before his own board by reports on the web.

Curing Cancer and All Disease the Easy Way

Your body can only heal itself. Cancer is but one expression of some form of a toxic overload. Take away the overload or the missing frequency and the body will generally heal. However, there are no spontaneous remissions with cancer. And drugs can never heal the body of any disease as their vibrations are isolated, targeted, and distorted of natural frequencies.

Cancer is but one of the many life threatening diseases. What sets it apart are the costs involved in its treatment and the fact that the quacks have been far more successful at actual cures than mainstream doctors.**http://www.cancerdefeated.com/newsletters/The-cancer-cure-that-mystifies-doctors.html**

However, given the above Quantum Science, no disease is beyond curing and none can be separated at the quantum level. That is, these are all frequency oriented problems and when the missing frequencies are reintroduced, by whatever means, such as removing toxins or replacing the missing essential frequencies the disease ceases to exist.

Thus, all diseases are curable as Dan Nelson discusses in his talks. That is, life threatening diseases go away when the correct vibrational qualities are met. With the new understanding of how vibrations affect us, nothing is impossible when it comes to cures and, from the opposite side, no one should become diseased in the first place. All foods are simply vibrations and essential minerals are essential vibrations. You can't be in harmony with missing vibrations, but these are not the only sources of these vibrations, only those most readily available to the general population.

While the above cancer cures may work (or not), herein, I give you a method that will cure any disease, quickly and in a proven way. When you accept this quantum healing premise, that all disease is frequency based and you see a disease immediately disappear when these balances occur, you simply know, and the results are indisputable. From this, we understand that until now, we have been looking in all of the wrong (complex) places for cures and no other is needed.

Diagnosing from Beyond the Sub-Conscious Level

While this ability is limited to a few individuals with adequate spiritual training, we see a time when those "ordained" and trained in these teachings and techniques become the true healers of the 21st century, a time when invasive disease diagnosis, will no longer be accepted or even allowed by society as awareness of these possibilities increases and the drug culture is abandoned. This stands in direct opposition to the current drug oriented medicine that claims that they can break down nature's herbs and chemicals, give them a name, patent them, and a doctor can implement them to cure you of a disease.

Our own claim is that the best that any drug can do is hold off the detrimental effects of a disease till the body cures itself. In most cases, we claim, that drugs can never go this far. Drugs serve mainly to relieve the pain and symptoms. This can cause more problems, since pain is an essential part of the body's defense system in that it warns you of impending problems.

Herein, we discuss "Cures," and not pain relief. Our methods are simple and they rely on building your autoimmunity through a powerful quantum blend of frequencies that include microorganisms and foods that can avoid the harmful parasites and diseases. This results in a healthy body that literally is always well, happy both mentally and physically and thriving in ways never seen on this planet for thousands of years,

As this cutting edge science of Epigenetics catches on and it is accepted it as scientific facts as it must, these healings will become far more common (once again). At first, they will be considered "spontaneous" by the drug culture, because in their minds, a drug or some outside intervention must be used to change a body grossly. This is not true and as time goes on, it will become common knowledge as it was thousands of years ago.

Quantum Healing (QH)

The actual quantum treatment side, especially when fractals are employed, is quite mechanical and scientific in its application, effects, and outcomes are 100% predictable once diagnosed. While these are no more spiritual in nature than healings have ever been, these healings and anti-aging methods depend on your definition of spirituality, since vibratory frequencies may certainly be included in that definition. The basic idea here is that everyone always has always healed themselves and this can never change.

Quantum Healing (QH) is the ultimate topic here. It incorporates all aspects of the new science, epigenetics (and beyond, as discussed above). The method of QH includes: fractals, fractals embedded in metals, monatomic metals and an individual program embedded in our lab crystal set (CP4U-F) (the very same crystals employed in microchip technology) used in tact and unaltered. These contain an induced program as selected by the healer to counteract the health concerns and thus raise the vibratory frequencies that identify the patient along with the fractal set, etc. These individual parts, when combined properly, produce profound healing effects previously unavailable. The final result is that not only are you healed of the offending disease, your cellular age is lowered, Telomeres are lengthened, and your microcellular energy factors are raised to levels previously unattainable. Thus, your body is literally driven to frequency levels unknown to modern man and you thus become a superhuman being with a far greater energy potential and life span.

Fractals

Historically, the most simple and commonly known fractal is the star of David, a two-element geometry comprised of equilateral triangles repeated and inverted. From this, we can expand them to complexities beyond all comprehension as the geometry expands as nature wills it. As a friend suggested as we discussed the Star of David: Do you think that they knew something in those ancient times? The answer, of course is: Yes, they did!

Fractals are the organizing principals of all of nature. They can scale up in both their geometry and in the energy patterns that they enhance or linear. They represent patterns of sound and light which, spiritually, are the highest, yet most simple, of organizing principals. In fact, fractals serve as filters of essentially the diagrams of harmonic frequencies. Thus, they are in no way chaotic as the current Newtonians teach. The reverse is also true. The fractals produced by any healthy biological entity are well organized and their frequencies are harmonically balanced and whole.

Thus, if we considered the Star of David as the organizing fractal of a biological entity that was ill, the star might be missing a point and would thus be unbalanced, disorganized and thus chaotic and highly energy consuming (like a leaky roof). Biological entities are, however, far more complex in their organizing harmonics than this most simple fractal.

The resulting harmonic from a healthy person might be comprised of fifty or more frequencies. If just one frequency is missing or low, the overall harmonic is unbalanced and discordant. This person is sick and thus consumes more energy and is less efficient as the body attempts to bring itself back into balance. This is then, a new definition for disease.

Fractals, when employed to heal, are generally balanced geometries that filter the harmonics and thus alter the vibrational tones when applying them to people. These, then, are the organizing principals that are optimally stacked along with monatomic metals so as to repair and offset the frequency and resulting energy losses that the subject disease is causing. Corrective foods and diets, which are also just frequencies, can create the same results, but they are slower acting and not as dramatic in their effect. We are in a constant search for a more powerful fractal combination for a particular discord.

What else has been forgotten and lost as modern science has trampled on what was once held as sacred, or is now considered as just subjective religion, and thus disregarded by it?

We have cherry picked Newtonian Science as the winner and dropped all aspects of the work done by alchemists, all the while complementing ourselves for our brilliance. Alchemists are now commonly considered as misdirected, even insane, sorcerers, who were said to be attempting to change cheap metals into gold. When misunderstood, it is easy to find fault, as the drug industry does with naturopaths, especially when it helps their pocketbooks.

So, given the above, verbally all of creation speaks with fractals, but they have been avoided by modern science, totally, until just the last few years. When employed in biological systems that have gone awry, the systems recompose with a new more powerful order. Thus, healings occur instantly and, moreover, health can be improved to levels never before seen.

Therefore, with this astounding fractal technology, the human body can be improved at the microcellular level to cure all disease, increase energy levels, and generally improve all aspects of life in ways previously unknown. Yes, this is being done today, but the cultural lag, as financed by the pharmaceutical and medical industries, we know, will attempt to hold it back. Incredibly powerful, nothing in modern times has ever shown the promise that these age-old notions provide, so the real question is, how long can these powerful controlling money systems hold back this powerful new science? Long term, quantum healing must win, in our opinion. People will get it and no amount of marketing can overcome the facts as they reveal themselves.

Interestingly, complex hydraulic, electrical and mechanical systems are improved to impossible levels when these patterns are applied to them also. When employed, these Quantum systems exceed all of the restrictive laws and limitations that are commonly agreed to and held as limitations by today's Newtonian science.

Our CP4U-F, being marketed today to increase internal combustion engines of all types, is likely the first modern era example of an infinite quantum fractal application. Thus, this is a breakthrough device that can be purchased and installed on your car. In the Egyptian Old Kingdom Era (lost over time) this was a commonly accepted method of doing work. In that era, this technology was used correctly and it accomplished most of the difficult and now considered, nearly impossible, work that was done in making and moving the massive, nearly perfect, stones in pyramid building. Pyramids themselves are totally misunderstood also. These were not just tombs, there were QE energy factories as proven by scientists like Dr. Patrick Flanagan who has written several books on how pyramids actually work and followed by many others since. These, of course, have been disregarded by the Newtonians also.

Nothing today in what is now called "modern science" or Newtonian Science can explain how the Egyptians actually moved those stones with such precision or, as with our CP4U-F, how energy output can increase as fuel use decreases. This CP4U-F technology, when understood, demonstrates that all dynamic engineering systems common today will be outdated eventually once these systems are adapted and we transition into this modern quantum era of healing and mechanics.

Definitions of Fractals that Miss the Mark

Per Google: (Fractals are) the infinitely complex patterns that are self-similar across different scales (referred to often as scalar below). They are created by repeating a simple process over and over in an ongoing feedback loop. Driven by recursion, fractals are images of dynamic systems – (Herein called) the pictures of Chaos. Herein, we suggest that Google misses the mark as most of today's science does. In fact, fractals only appear chaotic when misunderstood. Scalar energy systems work from the minute to the extremely large and, thus scale up, generally, just as our earlier CP4U once did. Today, the fractal versions can be flat and linear, scalar, or in combination as we select in our programs.

While the web is full of definitions and lectures on fractals by revered physicist (search them from Tom Beardon who reveres scalar energy and heard at: **http://www.cheniere.org/toc.html** to Bruce Lipton), nothing nor anyone out there can actually demonstrate the results reported beyond what Lipton indicates at

https://www.brucelipton.com/books/biology-of-belief
from direct experience, but we can.

Furthermore, there is very little second party verification
other than the survivors of Rich's beneficial healing
effects using this fractal technology, most of whom
currently have no voice that can be heard above the
thundering voice of drugs. So theories abound while
applications and results are currently not demonstrated on
a large scale thus far. Still, with the arrival of the field of
Epigenetics over the last ten years and the welcoming that
it has received, we expect a ground swell in acceptance as
the cards begin to fall.

Vibratory Frequencies

You are a unique set of higher vibratory frequencies
which together result in a single harmonic frequency.
This resulting harmonic is sometimes referred to as Soul
on the spiritual level. While this may be seen as spiritual
in nature and empirically, the frequency levels are
measurable and knowable from a quantum viewpoint. So
what the ancients were teaching is not only true, it is now
actually measurable and scientifically based.

For instance, Dan Nelson has found that frequency 28 is
always missing when a person is in a cancerous mode.
For a person to rise above this mode, this frequency must
be restored or eventually they will not survive. Cancer is
just one mode of survival that signifies a restricted total

harmonic level, so when one raises the harmonic level and it disappears. Thus the cancerous condition can come and go in seconds. The compromised cellular conditions that lead to it can take years to arrive at these levels, but your body turns it on in order to survive.

Dis-Ease

As repeated herein in several places, when the various frequencies that comprise an organic system are out of harmony, it is in a state of Dis-Ease.

In an animal, this disease can be expressed in anything from a common cold to the common life-ending diseases such as cancer and heart disease. These life-ending diseases are subjective names for missing frequencies, misalignments, and vibratory holes in our cellular systems that are commonly expressed as system failures.

All can be cured when the frequencies are brought back into balance or harmony in our case using a fractal grid along with various vibrational frequencies. Thus, there is no such thing as an incurable disease. While an imbalanced condition can be the result of years of dietary abuse or inadequate vibratory conditions, these can all be "cured" in minutes, yes minutes, when the body is subjected to the proper balancing frequencies and is thus harmonically balanced. This, I have witnessed occur

34

several times recently, even time reversals have resulted that changed outcomes.

Cellular Energy Systems/ Mitochondria

You are a complex system of organic microcellular energy systems. The most obvious set is occurring in the mitochondria, the organelles that supply your life energy and allow life to continue. Interestingly, when an animal dies, these organelles shut down in unison just as if the body has just flipped a light switch. Thus death is an agreement, of sorts, in every case. For people, when they are not well and have a long term energy problem, the mitochondrial count could be as low as 10 per cell and 100 is common at mid-life.

Raising the Mitochondrial Count

When the objective is to heal, as discussed, the average mitochondrial level correspondingly increases, thus the fractal set used, in its inherent wisdom, supplies a higher frequency level, thus causing them to multiply. This is just one form of long-term healing. Even when done properly, raising the average mitochondrial count to 2400, the highest level sustainable, takes months following the treatment. Most people are born with 700 to 800, but with this advanced quantum healing, this maximum 2400 level can be achieved.

35

The Implications of Quantum Healing

Ancient scripts like the Old Testament Bible speak of the ancients living to 800 years. The conditions that allowed this to occur included a level of hydration that today's water will not allow. We have Wayback Water as marketed by Quantum Physicist, Dan Nelson. This level can be temporarily raised by the fractal healing, but to maintain it, one must take Wayback Water on a daily basis and it is imperative for a healing to occur.

The Biological Subsystems

If the digestive system is inadequate and lacks the cofactors, the frequencies, even if otherwise available, will never be delivered and your body will simply starve, no matter what your food intake is. Today we know that you are not just a single animal, but a complex biological system that cooperates to keep you in harmony. These cofactors actually supply your cells with B vitamins and other cofactors that you are unlikely to ever obtain otherwise.

Thus by taking antibiotics you kill off this complex life-sustaining system of cofactors that for many years were not even recognized by so-called modern science. So taking antibiotics is just one way of short circuiting these necessary biological systems. Radiation events of any kind have the same effect. Thus, MRI or and X-ray

36

testing can set your biology into a downward spiral by killing off key parts and thus short-circuit the required optimum harmonic frequencies.

Diet

Dietary input is basically frequency input and the term "balanced diet" implies a frequency balance that results in an overall harmonic balance. When you deprive your body of essential frequencies, especially by missing what are termed as essential minerals, it becomes disharmonious. For more on this, listen to Dr. David Perlmutter:
http://www.drperlmutter.com/news/brainchange-david-perlmutter/

As discussed herein and in my previous books, especially, modern farming practices have deprived us of many essential frequencies. Thus, our society is commonly lacking the needed wellness frequencies and is thus disharmonious, unwell, and diseased. A quick search of the common life-threatening diseases will reveal that they occur more frequently than ever for this reason.

Keeping the Ideal Mix

Thus, with the entire above mix, the quantum healing system will suddenly allow recently unprecedented life spans to occur as long as the necessary frequencies and

37

cofactors are maintained on a daily basis. So how do you do this? Food, minerals, and 100% hydration rates, along with the vitamins, fats (especially cholesterol as my 1st book and Perimutter, above, points out) and enzymes required to supply them. All are simply frequency enhancements and nothing more, just as sugar generally works in opposition to them.

Adding too much of a single factor (over eating, even otherwise ideal foods like nuts or fruits) or eating negative vibrational foods like candy, packaged commercial foods, or sugar loaded drinks (even orange juice) will immediately short-circuit this process. These may not lower your body to diseased state immediately and it may recover if brought back in balance. However, doing this is additive and eventually will take its toll, lowering your vibratory rate to that of the norm, which means essentially that you will begin to fail as an organism at about fifty years of age and die at age 75 or thereabouts as dementia sets in and the various systems begin to fail permanently as discussed herein.

Telomeres

It has long been recognized that telomeres decrease in length with aging. Also, when scientists measure telomere length, they have determined that biological entities with shorter lengths of telomeres are more disease prone and thus all biological systems are more likely to break down allowing the person to die. Thus, the telomere link is associated with the biological aging clock as noted in the article below.

http://www.alsearsmd.com/ppc/PPC_FOY_proconly.h tml?utm_source=google&utm_medium=cpc&utm_ter m=ad&utm_content=buyer&utm_campaign=telomere _foy&gclid=Cj0KEQiAsdCnBRC86PeFkuDJt_MBEi QAUXJfLWTsDCPQocqkGCBJM_VhpGpsY1ePPdiJ z90rAGY3Os8aAoGg8P8HAQ

Interestingly, when the quantum healing protocol is employed, telomere length increases substantially along with mitochondria as discussed above. Nothing out there can compare to the increases obtained, but there are less effective methods of increasing telomere length and, no, supplementing telomerase will not do what quantum healing does, but it apparently could help. The bottom line is that teleomeres are a function of frequency rates and microcellular harmony, not the reverse, as these scientists propose. However, every aging factor studied thus far, as the above article indicates, has shown that longer telomere length is a direct indicator of health and antiaging, so it may not cause health as commonly attributed, but it is certainly an indicator

Now, moving along, I introduce recent online discussions involving more conventional issues as they relate to the quantum healing method:

Heart Disease and Packaged Supplements

Hi Frank:

>You said BBAC (Blockbuster All Clear) is one of the best ways (to clear up HBP), but there are others... so can you tell us what they are? Thanks<

Read the label. BBAC is a combination of supplements.

Heart disease (more correctly, circulatory disease), is really just hardened tissue fighting to keep working efficiently, & thus keep you alive. When it can't do that, it fails or parts fail, the chief problem being the pump itself, but also, the circuit becomes leaky from the pressure needed to pump high levels of blood through a brittle set of pipes. The high pressures need to make the system work at all eventually take their toll on the pump. It enlarges to compensate and eventually fails. This is our most common health problem leading to death with a projected 23.6 million death per year by 2030 if today's "prevention" systems remain in place per the AHA.

The Author takes these interventions regularly, avoiding sugars and grains as reported in , "It's the Liver Stupid." As Dr. Perimutter and other mainstream doctors slowly learn, substantiate, and join what was once a very small Coconut oil group ten years ago. Why not? These dietary changes work, while the AMA and FDA still resists them and push statins and low cholesterol and bad fats. They all make good sense when you read the chemistry and this is how your body was designed to function..

Also, when you take these separately, they are cheaper. They post the ingredients on their BBAC site. BBAC would be similar to taking a multivitamin. As you are a unique biological specimen, if you are really paying attention, your unique blend will surpass any commercial BBAC blend such as this, just as your combination of supplements will be far better than any multivitamin can be.

Realize that Duncan Crowe was (and is) a supplement salesman and he brought this to the table on line in our discussions and reports on BBAC on his website. However, I suggest that HL MSM will do what BBAC will do, given sufficient time and a low carb diet will simply add to it as will Undenatured Whey. That is, MSM will make all connective tissue supple so that your arteries and veins will become elastic and renew.

But eating just one plant every day is not a good idea and neither is relying on HL MSM alone. You take the full complement as I suggest and herbs with their magic phytochemicals are synergistic along with the fats. Personally, I take a gram of probably ten powerful South American Jungle herbs each day, a pile of methyl B's, D3, Undenatured Whey Protein Isolates, Lipo-C, minerals (esp. Mg & Iodine), plus the various components associated with the Methylation Pathways like GABA (Gamma Ammino Butyric Acid) a key contributor here. The real key to this is reading and learning about how these pathways work and helping them along.

The above pathways are complex, but they are universal. That is, while you are quite different in the way that these pathways play out, your microcellular level (quantum level) is virtually universal, except as noted herein. Where we mainly vary is in how we affect them, especially at the subconscious level (epigenetics) and dietary levels. This is discussed in"Methylation, Awareness, and You." This side of the story not disclosed during, "It's the Liver Stupid.". It is because of this aspect that you can be exposed to the very same destructive poisons as another and you can become cancerous, while they are unaffected.

What is claimed here is that cancer is a self protective mode and not really the terrible disease commonly thought. That is, the body uses high blood pressure as a preservation mode. Similarly, in that raising your blood pressure as a way to keep you alive by combating the hardened tissue and micro-blockages that have occurred as a result of mainly not feeding your body adequate organic sulfur, good fats, and other key ancillary foods.

However, what you supplement with is no doubt less important than the foods that you avoid. like sugar, potatoes, bread, fried foods, etc which lower you body frequencies. If you play tennis with twenty-year-olds, you have to be very careful with what you take in at age 73. The idea here is to grow wise as you grow old. In doings so, you effectively grow younger... even look younger in this process. Interestingly, as your body grows younger, so does your mental outlook. This is the process that Duncan Crowe suggested here ten years ago and what is laid out in the two previous books. Realize that growing young will create social problems and some people are just fine with aging and dying. This issue is discussed later herein in more detail.

Energy Cycles and Balances

>Hi Paula: I've tried drinking water with Celtic sea salt, but found it hard going. I watched this video and found a much better way, put a bit on my tongue and then wash it down with lots of water. I love this Aussie. I want to watch all her videos as she knows her science but she makes it so accessible.<
https://www.youtube.com/watch?v=emHO3NekWLw &list=PLX8vMw5EroQIhKVoXKOz9WYFjMGqmh LxL

You may love Barbara O'Neill (and she is indeed very clear in her videos). There is no problem with what she says, mostly. The problem is with what she leaves out. She is at least ten years behind the current science (as discussed herein). However, nearly every lecturer on You Tube today is ten years behind current science, So she is no exception. I will point you to some of the speakers herein, but the most up to date work all stems from the quantum healing referenced herein. If you are ill or bent on staying well, you really do have to grasp this science yourself. Barbara is not going to lead you to this level of understanding.

Yes, sea water is great stuff but mainly transdermally, as she suggests in her discussion. But swim in it and please don't drink the combination. The idea of drinking sea water is misconceived. Magnesium and organic sulfur are still very important in our health link and both must be supplemented in today's world.

Think about it: If drinking sea water were a good idea, sailors would never be concerned with drinking seawater or supplying freshwater on their rafts. They know that they will die if they drink it. This occurs for good reason. Her diagram of swelled cells occurs when seawater is consumed over am extended period.

As far as High Blood Pressure (HBP) goes: This woman is very good up to a point, but she could lead you astray on this issue also. HBP (as discussed elsewhere herein) is a natural reaction to eating poorly grown food deficient in organic sulfur. This is why HL MSM works so well. It actually softens your arteries and veins and lowers blood pressure. HBP is mainly a natural adjustment to hardened arteries and closed off capillaries which all cause circulatory problems.

Note: Vitamin D is not a vitamin, it is a hormone in that the body makes it from cholesterol. This is why the pros will warn you not to take too much D3. While the levels of excess D3 have been greatly overstated, one indication that you do not have enough is expressed as the common cold. So if you begin to get cold symptoms, just take more. 50,000 IU is easily within the risk factor of most of us and most can commonly take that much when a cold is felt coming on. Doing this commonly results in complete remission and you should never experience another one if you do this.

No one in our society is hydrated today. However, to become hydrated, drink Dan Nelson's water which is comprised of 3-4 nanometer sized particles. No other water is close to this when it comes to absorption rates. One liter per day of his water will keep you 100% hydrated. So Barbara's intake rates are very high, but are commonly overstated, since no one generally knows about Dan's water. Too much water flushes you of the electrolytes as she points out and these are electrolytes are a significant key to your health.

45

Barbara's diagram of cell mitochondria is deficient and here is why: Most of us are not even aware of just how many mitochondria each cell average (MCA) actually contains or why maintaining as high number is important to your energy levels and overall health. You were born with an average of 800 MCA. The numbers normally decreases as you age. A very sick person with terminal cancer will typically have as low as 10 MCA or less. A healthy fifty-year-old will commonly have 100 MCA. There are naturally higher concentrations in liver cells, because the liver is the key organ and it basically oversees all others, while skin cells will have the least mitochondria per cell.

However, we have consistently found that the maximum MCA attainable is about 2400 per cell. Also, when cellular frequencies are harmonically in balance, they increase over time. Normally, the aging process includes a decrease in the MCA and this is common. Since these are the mitochondria creates the body's energy, your mitochondria increases in direct proportion to available energy levels, while the aging process saps the body of available energy which we see as normal today.

The body's harmonics are balanced by optimal mineral balance or external sources. Can you optimize them just with supplementation? Probably not. Rich uses a "fractal stack" to do this in his healing. Fractals are the geometric filters of all biological harmonics as previously discussed.

46

Your circulatory system is a complex fractal (as are your nervious and lymphatic systems. If one maintains this 2400 MCA level, they can run for miles without being winded at any age, Dan Nelson suggests that he can do this on his video.

Barbara is correct on her evaluation of Migraines in that dehydration is, apparently always the cause. If you maintain 96% hydration or more, you will simply never have headaches or migraine attacks. When you become ill you expel electrolytes, this headache results from dehydration. Migraines are more complex, but hydration is the key to beating them in virtually all cases.

Barbara's surface tension lecture is mostly correct and much of what she reports on is highly studied by the Scientist Dr, Gerald Pollack and carefully presented in his book: "The Fourth Phase of Water."

However, despite Pollack's work and his eminent credentials, reducing surface tension is just not the answer to optimum hydration. This was also proposed by another of my other heros, Dr. Patrick Flanagan. But it is not the case. That is, Megahydrate, which does this, is just not the answer to 100% hydration. The Dr's Batmangelhedi **https://www.youtube.com/watch?v=oCfDzPs8tvA** and Emoto **https://www.youtube.com/watch?v=Is8FE0RQo8A** did

47

some fascinating work also, but neither ever came up with the real answer when it comes to true hydration as 100% cellular hydration no longer occurs in nature. The true reason is sourced again from the Quantum Scientist, Dan Nelson
https://www.youtube.com/watch?v=7hNW7qxIMzg
That is: water particle sizes today are just far too high. Until he invented his reverse-time laser which he uses to create his water, his 3-4 nanometer water was simply unavailable in today's world and we were, as he says, dehydrated. Now, maintaining full hydration is simple. Also, if you are ill, the fact is that nothing will make you fully well till you are 100% hydrated. That is, 100% hydration is just the starting point to vibratory balance and this is where Rich begins when he works with his quantum fractal healing.

Moving onto Barbara O'Neill's lecture on exercise:
https://www.youtube.com/watch?v=nlxkGzovuEU&index=2&list=PLX8vMw5EroQIhKVoXKOz9WYFjMGqmhLxL&spfreload=10

Frequency is a vibratory level and it is commonly expressed in hertz (that is, movements or cycles per second). It does not mean "done frequently" as Barbara implies.
This is a cute explanation as it relates to exercise, but it is misleading and the term is becoming increasingly important as we move into this Quantum Realm.

Certainly, Barbara has a way to go. However, if you are to achieve the levels of health suggested herein, you must not be confused by her above statement. In particular: foods, and minerals are simply frequency balancing elements. These element themselves close the frequency diagram if one were to draw it just as the Star of David is balanced and closed, but in a much more complex diagram. Furthermore, when an element is lacking, there is a fissure or leak in the Methylation Energy Cycle, the diagram is no longer balanced, and disease is commonly the result. Conversely, when complete harmony is achieved, wellness and anti-aging begin.

Exercise is important, but too much exercise, which is unbalanced, is simply stress, and stress of any kind will cause disease. The best exercise comes in bursts, now often termed as interval training, not just in walking or unstressed exercise, as Barbara suggests. The Mayo clinic describes it at:
http://www.mayoclinic.org/healthy-living/fitness/in-depth/interval-training/art-20044588

Everyone Should Stop Eating These Four Foods!

https://www.youtube.com/watch?v=x5gXRFfMS3g

Dr. Peter Glidden opens the interview discussing the growing number of anti-depressant prescriptions. The discussion leads to the reason for an increased organic mineral intake to prevent disease. This leads Glidden to his "String of Pearls " as discussed below.

This is a good explanation of why we are a sick nation, mentally and physically, The first to popularly tell about this was Dr. Joel Wallach of "Dead Doctors Don't Lie," now almost twenty years ago. Minerals are really the bottom line nutritionally, just as he told us then, but now we know that there is plenty more to the wellness and anti-aging formula than just minerals.

This is the String of Pearls that are so easily joined, they tell you why you are not well, even if you think you are. If you are eating the same foods as the general population, you are (all) basically sick, even if you are not yet aware of it. We have come to accept sickness as normal and discuss our warnings of illness with such terms as, "Its just Growing Pains," or the "Pains of Old Age." No, these are all indeed abnormal. Pain is simply your body screaming, "I am not well!" "Help me please, before I die." "Get me some proper foods with real minerals that I can use and restore the harmonic frequencies that I need to maintain my health."

Peter gives you a fun "gluten" test here that is going to teach you a lesson quickly if you take it.

Never be satisfied with pain reducing drugs as a solution. When you take them, you are telling your body, "Shut up and just live with what I am feeding you like everyone else." This is what our medical profession, the FDA, and drug companies have degraded us to. Their common term is "pain management." A proper diet, free of gluttons and complemented with a full range of organic, bioavailable minerals, will bring love songs to your body and you can throw away your aspirin and pain killers.

Optimum Body Weight and HBP

>The following link is an article from Life Extension Foundation about a high blood pressure medicine that has "significantly" lower side effects; but most important, has a number of longevity effects. Herein I summarize the important points in the article. However the article does contain a lot of history about high blood pressure medicine and references to trial, studies, etc. Also the article does point out that one should first deal with high blood pressure via diet and life style changes. When that fails to lower the blood pressure, a pharmaceutical drug may be the only solution in their opinion.
http://www.lef.org/Magazine/2015/3/Best-Drug-To-Treat-Hypertension/Page-01 <

With this, the question becomes the entire premise that your body does not recognize the correct blood pressure for your inner physical condition (i.e., the pliability and openness of arteries and condition of capillaries and veins). That is, if you have hardened arteries, your body adjusts as required. It must maintain a certain blood pressure to maintain the optimum level of health possible for your diseased condition.

Moving your blood pressure down to typically undiseased conditions is just an indication of ignorance of mainstream treatments. So, by this premise, lowering your blood pressure artificially is not a solution. What you really need to be doing is to soften up your entire circulatory system with the correct diet (per HL MSM herein), not adjusting the symptoms of the hardened dysfunctional system that your body is working feverishly to maintain a life force in.

As to the longevity effects: Body weight falls in line when you eat the proper diet. We all recognize that excess body weight indicates ill health. Fat eats your D3, arguably the most important source of health that you manufacture. The problem is to know what that weight is, since we are all different with no set health goals. However, one only needs to look at animals in the wild to see that none of the herd is ever commonly excessively fat or thin. They adapt or are eaten by carnivores. In our case, we just become diseased and die when we deviate too far from our optimum weight.

Parasites, Fungi, and Electromagnetic Devices

>In response to a CCO post discussing the Beck electromagnetic healing device not working<
>> The Comment: "Not noticing any benefit doesn't necessarily mean there is no benefit.

For instance, it would be possible to have parasites and be unaware that you have them, so you wouldn't be aware of them being zapped and gone ~ but having got rid of them, you would be spared later problems.

It's a similar story with supplements and superfoods, you may not feel any particular benefit, but they may well be keeping the body in balance and preventing disease.

The implication here is that the correct path is to listen to our intuition. There is a part of us that 'knows' ~ but we tend to override that with logic, outside authority, or general consensus.<<

Adding to the above: First off, assume that you have parasites because most people have some form of them and nearly all people have fungi of some form (closely related and often in combination). Moving from there:

First, the background: Our preoccupation with parasites took a big hit when the knowledge of beneficial gut bacteria came out in earnest starting in the 1990's. In fact, friendly bacterial are microcellular parasites of sorts and they are in fact key factors in your overall health and they make up a large part of your genetic structure. You have two or more pounds of them if you are healthy. So now we know that we are simply not alone as we assumed since Louis Pasteur passed on his radical antimicrobial ideas 150 years ago. He was wrong and now it is becoming more clear as time goes on just how far off base this man was in his conclusions. In fact, we now know that without correct bowel flora, you would be lacking in certain essential vitamins and, as Dr. Perimutter says: Your chances of getting dementia and Alzheimer's would go up considerably.

So, yes, you have parasites and some are beneficial bacteria, while others may be neutral and just stay in balance and cooperate with you without effect. We can now assert with confidence that everyone alive has microbes, fungi, flora and possibly even larger unknown parasites, yet all of these may be cooperating with your body and have no negative overall effect. The key to all of this is, or may well be balance and not eradication. But, of course, there are the parasitic diseases like Lymes and Malaria that kill. The bottom line is, as always, when healthy balance is lost, problems begin.

When you become ill, other bad guys move in and this is their expertise since all life attempts to prevail and thrive. These parasites occur with cancer and all major diseases as well as simple dynamic imbalances that occur from taking drugs and antibiotics..

With this in mind, you could theoretically overdo Beck's electrification devices. However, these Sota devices, in the hands of a talented, observant healer, can be awesome healing tools. The key is always in knowing when and where to apply them. In fact, it is quite likely that there is no benefit to be gained in killing off bacteria in many cases. The key is always balance despite what the brilliant Dr. Robert Beck believed in his day.

Histamines, Allergies and Natural Solutions

> Question: I get some histamine reactions, such as runny nose (right after eating certain foods). Is that different from a histamine intolerance? What is the origin of histamines? I become sleepy and have low energy and tiredness after certain foods. I tried natural antihistamine supplements: vitamin C and a few others, but sometimes I react to those and also to Benedryl. Yesterday, I had more nausea than usual, so I tried a homeopathic, which helped some. Then, my son noticed my low energy level and suggested eating to raise my blood sugar. That helped me feel better (still nauseous though). I can't always tell that I need to eat.<

Allergies are a common autoimmune reaction and they are common to a large segment of today's illness accepting society. Over the last hundred years, this segment has grown enormously. One explanation is that, as a society, we are simply too clean and our systems no longer learn to deal with what are now pathogenic bacteria and once were simply dealt with as we went through life (and in balance). So, this is just one of the many ways that our modern methods of dealing with health have backfired badly. In coping with these problems, as noted below, we can actually short-circuit our healthy food choices in an effort to avoid the effects of our lifestyles.

In an allergic reaction, a heterocyclic amine, $C5\ H\ 9\ N\ 3$, is released by mast cells when tissue is either injured or there is an allergic and inflammatory reaction, causing dilation of small blood vessels. This results in a smooth muscle contraction that can be quite unbearable in many cases as addressed in the question below. These can often be resolved through natural means with some diligence (also a little education on your part is required), but we are not likely to move back to the agricultural lifestyle that most people mainly lived a hundred years ago.

I suggest, especially given the recent study below, that high levels of MSM could relieve this over a long enough period and this is one benefit of adequate organic sulfur reintroduced into the diet at the levels that once were common just a hundred years ago. That is, the small blood vessels can be made more elastic over time with adequate sulfur stores, thus the muscle contractions should begin to disappear and finally disappear completely in due time. Realize that few currently know this to be true and we are working in a whole new area here, even though it has been reported by others who have looked into it. However, I am fairly certain that this is true for all. Even for those people who have the CBS genetic defect which could initially impede this relief (thus, saying that this will work for most people when employed over a long enough period). Another benefit related to this is that the gut may become more porous and thus increase your hydration rates, thus alleviate the dryness and coughs associated with these conditions. Therefore, adequate cellular hydration can be a huge asset here and as discussed earlier, few maintain them.

Allergy/ MSM Trial

While I have referenced sources that claim that allergies are alleviated by MSM. This trial using 2.6 gm/day, minuscule by HL MSM standards, serves to somewhat relieve MSM. Below I reproduce the report and comment relative to past findings using HL MSM. The point here is that if you have allergies and most people in our society today do. Thus, it sounds like we have an answer that does not include growing up on the farm and eating dirt like I did:

Trial"

*"In 55 persons with allergic rhinitis (stuffed nose from allergies) given 2600mg MSM supplementation in an open-label trial for one month, allergic symptoms and respiratory complications were reduced by day 7 with symptoms reduction increasing at day 14 (not much more benefit between day 14 and 30) with no alterations in plasma IgE and histamine when subgroups were sampled; the potency was approximately 20-40% symptoms reduction but was not quantified.[42]"***http://examine.com/supplements/Meth ylsulfonylmethane/**

The point here is that if 2.6 grams per day had some effect, two tablespoons per day or more should be awesome, given what we have seen when HL MSM has been used for other problems, you can expect an usually good outcome.

Again, your allergic or asthmatic condition is common to many in our society today. While there are other probable factors as noted above, this is another direct result of our current farming practices that have removed organic sulfur from our soils.

By restoring organic sulfur to the levels that we had before farmers commonly used these destructive fertilizers, these problems could be alleviated. It may take you a year or so to build back adequate stores of sulfur, but when you do, you can probably expect complete relief. The HL MSM protocol entails a gradual build-up of MSM till you are taking at least two tablespoons per day.

Also, since no heat is used in this delivery system you get all of the MSM and a quicker build-up than nature commonly ever provided.

To take it, scoop it in and swish it with water for a long period, then swallow. Together with alleviating or removing your histamine problem entirely, your general health should improve greatly as you balance your sulfur needs, but there are cofactors to consider also such as adding astaxanthin (hard to get except through supplementation), adequate magnesium (also hard to get, but cacao is a good natural source), and D-3 (adequate sunlight and cholesterol in the body) to mix.

Watch Dr. Stephanie Seneff's interview on You Tube **http://people.csail.mit.edu/seneff/** Few have a better handle on organic sulfur than Dr. Seneff, but she has no idea about the HL MSM approach in resolving it. Although she does mention MSM occasionally in her talks saying she knows nothing about it.

Seneff gives you a bundle of reasons as to why this MSM is so effective at allergy relief, but one that she does not mention came out in a recent report discussed by Mercola where they discussed that it helped to basically increase

59

the water absorption in the gut by softening the walls. Softening tissue is the commanding strength of MSM in all of its applications from arteries to knee tissue, so this make sense.

Histamines in Foods/ Benedryl
Note that the symptoms of a Benedryl are exactly as reported above and they include sleepiness, dizziness, drowsiness, confusion, weakness, ringing in the ears, blurred vision, enlarged pupils, dry mouth, flushing, fever, shaking, insomnia, hallucinations, and finally seizures if overdosed enough.

Alcohol combined with Benedryl may increase the drowsiness and dizziness... another reason you should not drink it in addition to the warning below. I always wonder why people never seem to either read or believe the manufacturer's revealed effects of these drugs. Do they somehow believe that the FDA is protecting them from drug companies?

The important thing here is that the common treatment and the foods to avoid in treating allergies and histamines are directly counter to the foods that keep us well and this is a pervasive illness today. So you must make a choice between the good foods for wellness and those that cause allergies and reactions.

Histamine is a biogenetic amine that occurs in various degrees in many foods. In healthy persons, dietary histamine can be rapidly detoxified by amine oxidases, whereas persons with low amine oxidase activity are at risk of histamine toxicity. Diamine oxidase is the main enzyme for the metabolism of ingested histamine. Histamine intolerance occurs when you can't breakdown the histamines in foods fast enough. It is now known that pickled foods, cheeses, avocados, mushrooms and beets are among the most healthy foods on this planet, so your attention, if you are to remain here for long must be in alleviating this histamine toxicity as soon as possible.

Initially, and as long as you commonly have histamine reactions, it is best to avoid alcoholic beverages altogether, especially beer, champagne and wine (the undistilled forms and commonly the least destructive). Also, generally avoid anchovies, avocados, cheeses, especially aged or fermented cheeses, such as Parmesan, blue and Roquefort, dried fruits such as apricots, dates, figs, prunes, and raisins, fermented foods such as pickled or smoked meats, sauerkraut, mushrooms, processed meats such as sausage, hot dogs, salami, sardines, smoked fish such as herring, pickles, pickled beets, olives, sour cream, sour milk, buttermilk and yogurt (especially if not fresh). So notice, in reading this list, these are the very foods are generally recommended for wellness and longevity? This is the reason, the histamine and allergy problems are, as mentioned above, a huge issue that short

61

circuits our efforts to stay young even though this is never discussed by mainstream nutritionists and especially the drug ads.

However, soured breads, such as pumpernickel, coffee cakes and other foods made with large amounts of yeast, spinach, tomatoes, vinegar or vinegar-containing foods, such as mayonnaise, salad dressing, ketchup, relishes, chili sauce are also on the list and many of these do not make our heath list. So all is not bad and there is no doubt that you must be avoiding bread and sugar if you are going to stay young.

We now know that you can naturally acclimate to the above with help from a naturopathic healer who knows this is the new field of epigenetics. Lipo C might help with this (not C), but there are many other natural ways, when you dig down, and some are as follows: Butterbur is a supplement available orally that can help. Mangosteen, a fruit extract supplement, usually sold in juice form or as capsules is also useful (read the label for sugar added). However, Quercetin is one of the best, as the following report by J. Herb Pharmcother suggests in 2003: and this should be on your supplement list above all others:

A water extract of a mixture of eight herbs (chamomile, saffron, anise, fennel, caraway, licorice, cardamom and black seed) was tested for its inhibitory effect on histamine released from rat peritoneal mast cells stimulated either by compound 48/80 or be IgE/anti-IgE. The effect of the herb extract was compared to that of the flavonoid Quercetin. The herbal water-extract inhibited histamine released from chemically and immunologically-induced cells by 81% and 85%, respectively; quercetin treated cells were inhibited by 95% and 97%, respectively.

The clinical results showed significant improvements of sleep discomfort, cough frequency and cough intensity in addition to increased percentages of FEV_1/FVC in patients suffering from allergic asthma, who used the herbal tea compared to those who used the placebo tea, so neither of these are an answer (as we would expect). Interestingly, coffee, our drink of choice in the US is looking better as a health drink, in moderation, every day as the reports come in and it may help somewhat with its caffeine contribution.

As these non-pharmaceutical reports are seldom funded, they are rare.

Still, when you listen carefully to what Dr. Stephanie Seneff tells us about organic sulfur there are adequate clues here, if you believe in the HL MSM Protocol to suggest that MSM is the way out of this long term. Hydration is always a key to any of these therapies, so keep that in mind, also.

Parasitic Diseases

Malaria

Wikipedia on Malaria:

"In Africa, where 90% of all cases occur, malaria is
estimated to result in losses of $12 billion USD a year
due to increased healthcare costs, lost ability to work and
effects on tourism. The World Health Organization
reports there were 198 million cases of malaria
worldwide in 2013. This resulted in an estimated 584,000
to 855,000 deaths.
http://www.cdc.gov/malaria/about/facts.html

**http://www.who.int/immunization/diseases/malaria/en
/**

Malaria is a preventable and treatable (*not really*)
mosquito-borne illness. In 2013, 97 countries had
ongoing malaria transmission. There were an estimated
207 million cases of malaria in 2012 (uncertainty range:
135 – 287 million) and an estimated 627,000 deaths
(uncertainty range: 473 000 – 789 000). 90% of all
malaria deaths occur in sub-Saharan Africa, and 77%
occur in children under five. Between 2000 and 2012, an
estimated 3.3 million lives were saved as a result of a
scale-up of malaria interventions. 90%, or 3 million, of

these lives saved are in the under five age group, in sub-Saharan Africa.

There is currently no commercially available malaria vaccine, despite many decades of intense research and development effort. The most advanced vaccine candidate against Plasmodium falciparum is RTS,S/AS01. A large clinical trial with 15,460 children is ongoing in the following seven countries in sub-Saharan Africa: Burkina Faso, Gabon, Ghana, Kenya, Malawi, Mozambique, and the United Republic of Tanzania." Note: The current falciparum RTS,S/AS01 trial results are indicating that it is 31-56% effective according to age.

Treating Malaria Case Study

Rich treated a friend using Quantum Fractal Healing and below is the case study which I participated in passively. The person treated's chronological age was just 30 years, but their cellular age prior to the treatment was 48. The Mitochondrial Count Average (MCA) stood at 100, which is common for a person of 48 and especially for an ill person. Within four hours after initial treatment, most associated symptoms were gone and by the next day, there were none. Two days after the initial treatment, the cellular age tested at 30 years and MCA at just under 2000! Today, it stands at that of an 8 year old and 2400 MCA and there have been no recurring events after three months.

65

The MCA corresponds to an energy level of 24 times what it was prior to treatment with a cellular age of 4x less than chronological age. This suggests a permanent cure in this case. That is, Malaria should remain a distant memory for this person. With energy levels this high and cellular age is low, the body will commonly resist all parasitic future infections. This, of course, will not be proven as fact for many years, but few people on this planet have or maintain this energy level.

Our tests indicate that once a quantum healing has occurred (at least at this point), cellular aging never occurs again, but time will prove out just how long this holds up.

This treatment was done using only the person's picture and permission, which is commonly all that Rich needs to do this Fractally-based quantum healing himself. Given that this was his first treatment for this infection, the efficacy rate for malaria is not yet known. However, given that the healing was nearly instantaneous, one could assume that the healing rate could easily stand at 100% for all malarial patients once the technique is taught in Africa.

Rich had never before treated malaria or these strains of parasites and was not sure that this could even occur, but I was fairly certain that his quantum healing technique would work for this application, so I ushered him into it and it worked better than we guessed.

The point me here was that malaria is not so much different than the various Lymes Disease strains and associated parasite which this technique has cured routinely. We both learned a great deal from this healing in terms of its associated social implications as noted above from web searches. Malaria is perhaps even more socially disruptive than Lymes, but this is a difficult call since Lymes comes in so many variations and is not so recognizable as malaria.

My personal interest is in cancer curing which Rich has done successfully using his quantum healing (along with Alzheimer's to some degree), but we need more cases to make the strong case that this has made with Lymes and Malaria. The long term implications of all of this, are, of course, beyond belief. With each healing, we see the same associated anti-aging qualities that accompany the healing, as the MCA is commonly up 24x each time. My theory is that these techniques kill the associated parasites and the cancer goes away. That is, eradicate the detrimental flora (or the poison that created it) and the body will retract the cancer.

Our current interest will be to train a few thousand other practitioners to use Rich's fractal models and setup according to our methods and hopefully, eventually cure all known diseases, especially pathogenic varieties like Lymes and Malaria, which currently evade all know mainstream drugs once they are entrenched.

Lymes Disease

> Below is a comprehensive article on the Lyme—MS hypothesis from the CCO Group:
http://owndoc.com/lyme/multiple-sclerosis-is-lyme-disease-anatomy-of-a-cover-up/<

Watching her video, I have to ask, where is the "hook?" Diet and lifestyle are certainly important, but we know that many of our foods today have no productive content and that is probably the second main reason that we fall ill.

First, we now know, through epigentics, that all diseases are mental but we also know through Dr. David Perimuter that diet. Doctors have often hidden behind this as a diagnosis in the past, but with no scientific basis. So, most disease and illnesses set in due to negative influences in our lives after we have had dietary insufficiencies over a number of years. We have known this for years, but this new science tells us why and also that we can affect a cure using this fact. So few doctors today have an objective scientific basis for the fact that diet, lifestyle, and the sub-conscious mind are the actual causes of virtually all diseases.

68

MS is probably one of the most curable of chronic diseases. However, there are at least ten conditions commonly mistaken for Multiple Sclerosis making it one of the most mis-diagnosed diseases on the planet. Also, we now have many strains of Lymes running through our population as noted below (with people living in the Bronx contracting it through ticks on pigeons) that mimic MS. So MS is not a viral disease, but we have these advanced strains of Lymes that literally defy all common means of diagnosis, thus make people are diagnosed with MS. Some forms, as noted below, even include a viral strain that can never be detected by MRI.

Quoting Healthline:
http://www.healthline.com/health/multiple-sclerosis/new-diagnostic-criteria#2
"Magnetic resonance imaging (MRI) <u>cannot diagnose MS</u>, but it is the imaging procedure of choice for confirmation and to monitor the progression of the disease in both brain and spinal cord. MRI is the most sensitive imaging modality for diagnosing MS in the spinal cord, evaluating the extent of disease, and following response to treatment. It is more sensitive for identification of active plaques than clinical examination or CT scanning. <u>However, is it not specific for MS.</u>"
.

Diet and lifestyle are not likely going to cure Lymes once the Lyme borreliosis bacteria is contracted, but certainly they may intervene in keeping one from contracting it through epigenetics and immune defense.

Once contracted, doctors have no treatment for Lymes except massive anti-bacterials which cause all sorts of bowel problems when administered and, long term, must make it worse as our immune system is compromised and other diseases fall in behind it. Also, it is now known that at least one strain of bartoniosis (there are nine new known strains that elude all tests as noted below) is accompanied by the Powassan Virus. So what would you expect to happen when you treat a virus with massive doses of anti-bacterials? They drive them deeper only to have them return in five or ten years with a vengeance, with deadly results, and often on diagnosis.

MS is a totally curable condition, but it requires more than a correct diet and lifestyle in most cases. That is, you start with diet, lifestyle, and total hydration and move from there. You simply can't be totally hydrated by drinking tap water with its large molecules. As Dan Nelson says, we need water that will cross the cellular (EZ) barrier at .5 nm in particle size. Right now, we only have one source (WayBack Water), that can accomplish that, so most people are stymied right out of the gate and generally progressively deteriorate.

Lymes Strains

Currently, it is known that there are many strains of Lyme worldwide and it will continue to mutate frequently. As stated above, it is now diagnosed as MS, ALS, AIDS, Rheumatoid Arthritis and any number of other chronic diseases. Please read the report on this from "Common Cause Research Foundation:"

http://www.rense.com/general43/kly.htm

The bottom line is that if you are diagnosed with a neuromuscular disease, you must get second opinions and carefully evaluate them all, because Lymes can hide and not be detected at all. The clinical diagnosis, then, begins to look like many other diseases. Below of the currently known strains today and with new ones coming, often as we attack them with anti-biotics, which cause them to mutate into new vanities:

- Borrelia Afzeli,, Europe
- Borrelia Bissetti, US (mainly California and Illinois/ tests negative to standard tests)
- Shelter Island Strain (main US test strain)
- Kettle Forrest Strain (tests negative)
- Wisconsin Strain
- Borrelia Brugdoreri, US
- Borrelia Garinii, US and Europe

- Borrelia Valaisiana, Russia and China

RF (Relapsing Fever) Spirocetes RF is sometimes distinct for Lymes:

- Borrelia Hermsii, California
- Borrelia Miayamoyoi, California
- Borrelia Miyomotoi is more like Lymes than the others.
- Borrelia Parkcri, California
- Borrelia Pasturella, Egypt and Italy

In California alone, there are nine varieties of Bartonella that are negative to all other tests.

The Powassaan Virus is a flavivirus, a genus that also includes the West Nile virus, dengue virus, tick-borne encephalitis virus, and yellow fever virus. It transmits in 15 minutes time and is deadly.

So all of the above are potentially from one tick bite that usually transmit in 24 to 48 hours.

Treating Lymes

The same procedures are used for Lymes and Malaria and the results generally are generally equally good.

The Social Aspects of Wellness and Anti-aging

With all of this good news, as with all good things, there are some negative aspects to this quantum healing and some will eventually become profoundly earthshaking to those who depend on current methods and drugs which have no relevance in this newly uncovered advancement. The first warning of this coming, for those unaware, was epigenetics, which, if you are paying attention, proves scientifically that so-called modern medicine is doomed. As others learn this technology and it takes the place of these billion, even trillion dollar industries that have never really kept us well, what can we expect? More specifically, what are the social aspects of this as we move forward in this 21st Century? This is the big question that no one can really answer until those moments arise.

First, at the individual and family level, what happens when you elect to follow this new paradigm resulting in a much longer lifespan than commonly occurs and your spouse is unwilling to pursue it?

When your spouse announces, "I just want to grow old and die like the rest of society always has. Do you realize that you must go on alone? Realize that retiring, becoming sick and dying like everyone else is not where you are headed when you are a twelve year-old at the cellular level. So what are the reprocussions?

Obviously, in choosing this path, your needs are going to be very different and you must entirely reevaluate your life at some point. You might ask, "Is it OK to just leave and find a like-minded person even though you love your spouse?" Or you might just stick it out and painfully watch the people that you love, die. To do anything against their will and contrary to their wishes is spiritually incorrect. While it may not be the same as murder to disregard their choice, it is very nearly the same and no quantum healer will knowingly work with you to heal a person against their will. So this is a serious conflict.

Let's say that you are in your mid-seventies, normally within ten years of death and at a time of health breakdowns in today's society. You test out as age twelve at the cellular level, and your energy levels are through the roof. Your mitochondria count averages 2400 and have none of the degenerative physical problems common to your age group (or your spouse's) for obvious reasons.

What do you do? First, you must make one of the two choices and there is no other way. All others in your social network who avoid your choice will also pass on and you will be forced to find new friends and associates and socially adjust.

Taking the above into account, on an individual level, how should you plan and reorganize your life once you know that you will not be dying anytime soon. Will you find multiple new skills? Should you go back to school and learn a new profession, broaden your knowledge

74

base? Maybe you combine several skills and professions, knowing that society is bound to change as it picks up on these new possibilities.

Obviously, the healthcare industry in its present form is going to suffer some mighty blows as the need for managed care evaporates, the drug industry dissolves, and the medical professionals change to incorporate a degree of spirituality for the first time in anyone's knowledge today.

This trillion dollar industry, is going to suffer a huge setback as wellness displaces illness as a way of life. Just the fields of oncology at its current $70 billion a year cost and pain management at $60 billion a year will change the face of how both the providers and the patients live.

When people finally realize that antibiotics are killing their intestinal flora and refuse this method of treatment, then refuse most other drugs as an option... when their bodies are so healthy and immune systems so strong that they no longer normally become infected or even affected with pathogens... Where will this lead?

When the public commonly supplements the necessary levels of nutrients so that it no longer even becomes hypertensive and heart disease is a memory... What then? What will our attention be drawn to as a society when our future outlook is to deal with three hundred or even eight hundred years of wellness?

On a broader level, how will governments adapt as their social services become unnecessary and no longer required? How many years will it take before they realize that the services that they now provide are just needless expenses? If our average age suddenly (judging by historic standards), becomes 300 years, how will people cope with wars that wipe out large segments of our population of young people as they have over the last thousand years? Will war be tolerated at all with this new paradigm?

How long will it take before our entire legal system, based on life spans of around 70-80 years, adapts to the new paradigm? How will laws change to protect us from accidental death when essentially, this is the only way that people normally die? Finally, What new industries will emerge to encompass our new social needs and expectations?

So these are the problems and questions that we must deal with as we move forward. This new paradigm will and is already beginning to raise these questions for the first time in my own head(in apparently thousands of years) as we enter this new era.

Of course, these social questions will become far more prevalent and profoundly applicable as time goes on and these new quantum healing principles become more available and known. These questions predict that all basic social mores, that is, habits, manners, and attitudes are all about to be questioned (and many time dropped) as new ones displace our long held social values and needs.

So be ready as the current methods of relieving symptoms and pain, rather than healing, health, and anti-aging comes upon us. As those around you buy into this new paradigm and benefit as we have already seen only a few hundred or so at this point, you will learn to take these questions and outlooks seriously. For now, it sounds like a dream or wish.

Updating the HL MSM Protocol:

HL MSM... New Studies and Facts
http://articles.mercola.com/sites/articles/archive/2013/03/03/msm-benefits.aspx

First, I disagree with Rod Benjamin's marketing program and I do not agree that his more expensive product is necessary, or as good as cheaper crystalized MSM brands aimed at animals which is not denatured by heat. This report reminded me of this one key argument that I had forgotten in my earlier books:

But the first condition was always to use a product that moves quickly. Slower moving, more expensive products pick up more toxic elements in their manufacturing process and especially, storage.

The two MSM brands meant solely for human use employ the more expensive distillation process, as Rod Benjamin proudly reports, thus is by definition, denatured. Mercola agrees that this sounds like the better option till you understand that heat (or denaturing), destroys organic sulfur (and he was told this years ago as I document below)>

So this second reason for avoiding the expensive MSM is even more important to my HL protocol. This is, that the heat is used in the distillation of OptiMSM, Benjamin's company's process and thus has detrimental effects on the sulfur just as the farmer who gave me this protocol outlined years ago.

While the crystallization process may be dependant on the manufacturer's water quality as Benjamin says, and, yes, it could contain some contaminants if short cuts are taken. However, the key here is to find a solution that does not take shortcuts. As it turns out, most MSM end products actually test very well. But in picking your brand, read their data and follow the first rule above.

Finally, given the levels of use in the HL MSM Protocol, the product price difference is not pennies per dose since we actually use many times what Rod suggests or is even are aware of. That is, OptiMSM at between two tablespoons and ½ cup per day becomes significantly more expensive. Also, as reported in the earlier video, the MSM must be crystaline and "dirty enough to work."

While MSM occurs in raw milk, wine, veggies, tea, coffee, etc., Benjamin and Mercola both fail to mention, or do not know the following: Dr. Stephanie Seneff, who does not know (or did not know) about MSM (as she admits), clearly points out in her early interviews with Mercola that the heat of cooking and pasteurization remove the organic Sulfur from foods. Listen to her creative thoughts if you have not at: **https://www.youtube.com/watch?v=5QUChSlUEH0** Seneff is a wizard in many areas and her interviews are always very informative, search them all, but start here with this very long seven part series if you have not heard them. These touch on many aspects of health where we have gone badly wrong in the last hundred years.

The bottom line then: is buy bulk AniMed and the other cheaper brands designed for horses, as long as their quality control is maintained as recommended earlier in our HL MSM Protocol. Many seen to miss this point.

79

Notice that Benjamin does mention how raw vegetables do contain more sulfur, and this, per the above, this is absolutely true. The three reasons for our missing sulfur, as Stephanie Seneff in her interviews points out, are:

- We commonly cook our vegetables.
- Farmers employ sulfur killing inorganic fertilizers.
- Our diets lack cholesterol.

In these new studies, they discovered that MSM was indeed dose-related, but interestingly, this is was inversely related (?). That is, the more MSM you take, the less sulfate is excreted in your urine. This paradox may take a very long time to explain, but it is true.

This should raise the hair on your neck. What this says is that MSM is not just a strict sulfur donor as Rod points out and I reported in my last book. Of course, both Benjamin and Mercola need to study the methylation pathways as pointed out in my 2nd book, "Methylation, Awareness, and You."

These Pathways clearly indicate just how important the two methyl groups in MSM are as well as how sulfur contributes to the energy pathways at the microcellular level.
http://examine.com/supplements/Methylsulfonylmethane/

Realize, at this point, that increasing MCA is synergistic with the HL MSM effect and all of these health interventions create a snow ball effect that change everything at the micro-cellular level. As noted below, not only do these add to the picture, the picture even become more explosive as follow:

"It is a compartmentalization of sulfur and sulfur metabolism within the body. " This suggests, as Mercola points out, that MSM is actually creating better metabolism and better absorption of metabolites in general throughout the body. MSM is not just a simple sulfur donor. No, it is again the two methyl groups that do this, not the sulfur as I have pointed out all along since studying the pathways and relating them to the results reported.

As time goes on and other report on organic sulfur more outrageous results continue that literally defy medicine **https://www.youtube.com/watch?v=-EomFM8J3kk**, but these pathways begin to create an even more lively story the MCA is 2400 and it is combined with Wayback Water and none of this is know in the above interview,

Per Benjamin: New research determines "that approximately 15 percent of any DMSO dosage, on average, converts to MSM in the human body." Dr. David Gregg, PhD as I reported in my first book disagrees with these sparse results, it is much higher in humans. Rabbit studies are of little interest when it comes to testing MSM because their diets are totally vegetarian (correctly) and they do not suffer from our deficiencies.

Thus, the above conclusions need much more study, but these reports will be slow in coming. In fact, the conversion could be far closer to 100% per Gregg's observation, but these microcellular Methylation energy pathways (that the brilliant, late Dr. Gregg was likely unfamiliar with), are incredibly difficult to study objectively and time will tell. Furthermore, please note that, thus far, all studies and experts have underestimated every aspect of this HL MSM Protocol, so why expect them to be correct here?

This, I found to be the most interesting part of the above report and the part that Duncan Crowe and all government studies disputed till now (Crowe, because it competed with his Whey Protein Isolates Protocol results).

Most importantly, as reported here, MSM helps protect against "oxidative stress" and this is a key to anti-aging, our undisputed goal. Sulfur plays an important role in the production of Glutathione and this is absolutely the master antioxidant that your body produces as most experts agree. This detoxifies us of oxidants, poisons, and frees the Liver of stress allowing it to function at its optimum and thus helps keep you out of the cancer mode.

No, without sulfur, Glutathione clearly cannot work, per the pathways, a given. This is the key piece as agreed by the experts as we advance in this micro-cellular education process.

While not an antioxidant itself, MSM improves your body's ability to make Glutathione and other antioxidants. Thus, for detoxification, MSM is the most important antioxidant "effect" that your can ingest. So sulfur affects the body's master antioxidant resulting in lowing aging rates (and more so than any other single nutrient). Telomere lengths may also trump Glutathione. Till now, no one could alter telomeres or MCA rates, so neither were a consideration in this play. However, now we increase both through quantum healing techniques. The three, undoubtedly, combine to provide anti-aging levels never before considered.

Per Rod Benjamin (and all antioxidants go through these states): "Without sulfur, Glutathione has two different states within your body. There are reduced glutathione and oxidized glutathione." The ratio of those two signifies the overall oxidative state and the ability of your blood plasma to address oxidative stress. Also, keep in mind that this occurs at the microcellular level and mainly in the liver, which is why the liver has the highest levels of mitochondria in your body.

Per Benjamin: "MSM improves the above overall ratio by reducing the amount of the oxidized glutathione." In other words, without MSM, glutathione cannot do its job with the free radicals. At HL, MSM, as reported previously, thus becomes a super food. And yes, both MSM and DMSO do the same thing as they cross pollinate (per Dr. Gregg in my 1st book).. They control oxidative stress and protect against oxidative damage, thus we all benefit from their therapeutic benefits.

The above discussion, I previously discovered, predicted, and reported from my studies of the pathways on my own and others have verified in their own health benefits over the past ten years is in our various online discussion groups. That is, even without our past evidence, this HL MSM Protocol is all that I have claimed all along, if these new reports are correct and a good deal of evidence appears to substantiate that thus far.

We only need the real case study and confirmation as I have pointed out since my book. " It's the Liver Stupid" as first written in manuscript format some five years ago. But we now have some vague outside confirmation even if it is not directly applicable as follows:

Within the last two years, at least four clinical trials have proven, low level MSM has the ability to help with exercise recovery. Furthermore, muscle injuries like delayed onset muscle stiffness and soreness and "large muscle injuries like that from a heart attack" (all of which are related to oxidative stress and subsequent cellular damage) have now been substantiated, but this is just a start.

Clearly, sulfur and the two methyl groups in MSM affect sulfur metabolism at the cellular and microcellular levels as previously reported in my Book, "Methylation, Awareness, & You". This above report reinforces this idea to some degree. However, I suggest that the Methylation pathways clearly point in this direction and both Benjamin and Mercola must study these to understand why the results that they report are occurring.

MSM Toxicity Studies... More on the Above

As I have reported since 1999, the industry has no clue as to how well HL MSM or how fast most can progress on the HL Protocol without problems. In fact, for except those few with certain genetic problem, there is no toxicity, period. As others have reported, it is less toxic than water and the only real concern is with a Herxheimer reaction from releasing toxic build-ups. Below they tell you:

"Studies have shown that MSM is extremely safe and can be taken at very high doses." This is correct; however, I suggest that these writers are very naive as to what levels are most effective. They state:"Even if you have a very

85

rich diet, full of raw vegetables, and sulfur-rich foods, you can still supplement and not hit a toxicity level." But they are still discussing rates well below the therapeutic levels needed to actually cure arthritis, asthma, and circulatory disease per the statement: "Clinical research studies have found that the effective amounts range from about 1.5 grams to 6 grams." The point here is that clinical studies even at this late date miss the mark.

Keep in mind that members of our online groups commonly reach these recommended effective therapeutic amounts of two tablespoons a day or more within a matter of weeks, but some are far more conservative and have taken a year to reach these levels. Unless you have a great deal of pain, there is no problem with being this conservative, but we are all different and these few must use care.

However, for the rest of us, three grams/day is not even a start and six will generally do nothing for people over fifty. But yes, as they state, "All detoxifying effects can be minimized by cutting back on the dosage and slowly working your way up." My advice has always been to start at a level teaspoon per day and after a week without problems, double it and so on. There have been two reported problems in our groups (comprised of 4000) over a four year period and several actually reported starting as I did at two tablespoons a day with no harmful effects.

The HL MSM protocol is all about taking crystalized MSM loosely and orally, using what is described as swishing, not tablets. Furthermore, as discussed above, there can be no profound results at the normally discussed levels. However, the very young are the exception as their absorption rates are generally higher and those under age 25 can often do well on a few gram tablets. The point here is that older people just can assimilate enough to get well until they have been on the protocol for many years. Today, I generally do fine on a tablespoon per day at age 73.

Mercola ends saying that "People who might want to consider using some supplemental sulfur sources such as MSM include those who have:

- Chronic inflammatory conditions
- Aches and pains/sore muscles and achy joints
- Premature aging symptoms
- Toxicity"

Mercola's list is ridiculously short. I previously included several lists in my books that are probably five times as long. With HL MSM Protocol these are extended to include curing life threatening conditions like: HBP and Heart Disease, and even Mesothelioma in one case.

But Mercola is still learning and I give him credit for putting his report out. He is a leader in this industry, also, his suggestion that astaxanthin be taken with (HL) MSM makes sense and this agrees with my theory that MSM works synergistically with many other supplements.

So the above video is very informative even if Rod Benjamin is somewhat biased. As long as the person interviewed sells the product, one cannot expect an unbiased report, but he has pointed out some interesting facts from the new studies that we needed to be aware of.

Moving from people who obviously are at least open to the above reports, let's now look at some of the less open as follows:

The Quackery of MSM

http://www.quackwatch.com/01QuackeryRelatedTopi cs/DSH/msm.html
It is always of interest to look to Dr. Stephen Barrett for the most negative of all possible viewpoints when it comes to alternative and new science. He has always been the voice of negativity and the protective, entrenched viewpoint of the pharmaceutical industry, his supporters.

His Bottom Line: "No published research studies link MSM to any of the health claims made by its marketers. Sulfur needed in human metabolism comes from dietary protein (?). MSM supplements probably make little or no contribution to the body's sulfur requirements. Thus, there is no good reason to use MSM supplements."

Per the Mayo Clinic (a *less entrenched viewpoin*t), when discussing toxicity:

"Animals observed for 90 days on a daily dose of MSM five to seven times greater than what's typically used in people had no serious problems. Stomach upset, diarrhea and headache have been reported in human trials of MSM lasting up to 12 weeks. However, people taking a placebo also reported similar symptoms *(note that this last statement neutralizes claims that MSM is a toxin)."*

"Since little is known about the long-term safety of MSM *(given their references)*, it's no surprise that the efficacy also is unclear. Some studies of low level MSM have shown slight improvements in arthritis symptoms, but these studies were small and short term, so no definitive conclusions can be made."

In summary: As long as they rely on animal studies, low levels of supplementation, and the pharmaceutical industry for their results, clearly, no headway will ever be made in terms of this HL MSM Protocol (animal studies that make no sense in light of why it works as noted above). Still, the word is getting out as reported herein as follows. First, the most negative of the new reports:

PubMed MSM Trial Report

http://www.ncbi.nlm.nih.gov/pubmed/16309928
Our experience is that at this 3 gram/ twice a week level, virtually no significant results can be expected. However, this trial teaches us just how deficient most people are when it comes to organic sulfur. Furthermore, Rod Benjamin's observations based on this and the Bergstrom Study that follows are very creative, especially his insight gained from the MSM in urine samples.

Efficacy of methylsulfonylmethane (MSM) in osteoarthritis pain of the knee: a pilot clinical trial:

Authored by: Kim LS1, Axelrod LJ, Howard P, Buratovich N, Waters RF.

Abstract:

Objective:
Osteoarthritis (OA) is the most common form of arthritis and the second most common cause of long-term disability among middle-aged and older adults in the United States. Methylsulfonylmethane (MSM) is a popular dietary supplement used as a single agent and in combination with other nutrients, and purported to be beneficial for arthritis. However, there is *(a)* paucity of evidence to support the use of MSM.

Methods:
A randomized, double-blind, placebo-controlled trial was conducted. Fifty men and women, 40-76 years of age with knee OA pain were enrolled in an outpatient medical center. Intervention was **MSM 3g** or placebo twice a day for 12 weeks *(6g/day total)*. Outcomes included the Western Ontario and McMaster University Osteoarthritis Index visual analogue scale (WOMAC), patient and physician global assessments (disease status, response to therapy), and SF-36 (overall health-related quality of life).

Results:
Compared to placebo, MSM produced significant decreases in WOMAC pain and physical function impairment ($P<0.05$). No notable changes were found in WOMAC stiffness and aggregated total symptoms scores. MSM also produced improvement in performing activities of daily living when compared to placebo on the SF-36 evaluation ($P<0.05$).

Conclusion:
MSM (3g twice a day) improved symptoms of pain and physical function during the short intervention without major adverse events. The benefits and safety of MSM in managing OA and long-term use cannot be confirmed from this pilot trial, but its potential clinical application is examined. Underlying mechanisms of action and need for further investigation of MSM are discussed.

Bergstrom Nutrition Research
http://www.bergstromnutrition.com/our-
innovations/our-research/joint-health

Comments relative to the above study conclusion:

Three grams twice a daily does not comprise a sensible trial, so their meager results are to be expected.

The type of MSM used in the above study was distilled OptiMSM, so as previously noted, nothing about it fits well to the HL MSM Protocol as presented first in "It's the Liver Stupid.". This was funded by Bergstrom Nutrition and they sell OptiMSM. It did use 6 gm per day or seven times the PubMed levels, so one could expect far better results. However, the real problem here is that this study was done on "rabbits." As we all know, rabbits do not eat their vegetables cooked. Thus rabbits get organic sulfur in their food normally unlike humans. Finally, as discussed elsewhere herein, this was a distilled product, so much was lost as the organic sulfur content was greatly lacking.

Please now read "Non-metallic minerals"
http://www.beyondveg.com/tu-j-l/raw-cooked/raw-cooked-2h.shtml

From the above, I quote the following:

"Sulfur: Two important sulfur-containing amino acids, methionine and cysteine (both found in many plant foods, see Giovanelli [1987]) survive--to a large extent--after cooking. See Clemente et al. [1998] and Chau et al. [1997] for two research papers reporting the survival of these amino acids with cooking.
"Note that although there is some loss of sulfur-based amino acids in cooking, they claim the cooking makes minerals inorganic, if it were true, would require (nearly) 100% loss of methionine and cysteine. As that does not happen, these two common amino acids are.... etc.

Realize that HL MSM is a new protocol and no studies have been done on it, so we are in new territory at the moment. Dr. Seneff and I agree that Organic Sulfur is basically destroyed by any heat source over 140Deg F, which means that eggs fried hard are no longer a healthy source on sulfur. (However, she had no comment on this when I asked her about it recently)..

Heating Organic Sulfur

Below is probably the closest that one can get to the scientific detriments of heating organic sulfur today is as follows:
https://books.google.com/books?id=0zDNBQAAQBAJ &pg=PA200&lpg=PA200&dq=Heat+destroys+organi c+sulfur&source=bl&ots=FiaKOGBs- 4&sig=WPH4P6FESX5nQrncAdZsSdE4fqU&hl=en& sa=X&ei=cu0mVaHEH4risAWev4CoBA&ved=0CEU

Q6AEwCQ#v=onepage&q=Heat%20destroys%20org anic%20sulfur&f=false

I quote the following from that:

"We find that organic sulfur is reduced nearly 100% by all of the distilling methods attempted. "
Admittedly, they are vague as to their methods, but they are not discussing coal, yet two methods appear to be very high temperature.

There are purely chemical methods and two are quite powerful, so one might argue that they have no relationship to how they are handled in digestion by a human body and that is true. However, I suggest that distillation is always a powerful method of breaking down organic sulfur and if you are interested in keeping the sulfur in the MSM, temperatures greater than 140deg F must be avoided at all cost. This being the case, my initial warning when I wrote my first book to avoid distilled brands still holds.

Adding to this, distillation is commonly employed to reduce the sulfur in coal and this is the is the industrial focus of most studies. I am not suggesting that Bergstrom uses 1100F temps to distill their MSM, but you can be certain that their distillation exceeds the boiling point of water and is far above 140Deg F. Again, HL MSM is a whole new and relatively untested protocol at this point, but I suggest that Bergstrom money cannot change the facts. Eventually, as my protocol gains momentum just as my books continue to increase in sales, expect more real and unbiased studies to appear. The fact that somewhat mainstream sites like the one below now endorse at least the levels that I have taught for seventeen years, you can expect more rationality and objectivity in what we hear. However, just as with mainstream drugs, Bergstrom has the advertising power and they will be heard first for quite some time.

Sourcing High Level MSM

The most controversial aspect of the High Level MSM protocol that I introduced in my first book, "It's the Liver Stupid" has been with regard to the clarity of the product This is due to Bergstrom's claims directly related to the process used to oxidize MSM from its parent product known as DMSO or (CH3)2SO. DMSO can be oxidized by various mild chemical sequences in very high yields. DMSO is miscible in a wide range of organic solvents as well as water and has a high melting point. DMSO, itself, is produced from dimethyl sulfide, a byproduct of kraft paper pulping.

The chemical sequences, DMSO>MSM are outlined on the following two websites: **http://www.organic-chemistry.org/chemicals/oxidations/dimethylsulfoxide. shtm** and **https://www2.chemistry.msu.edu/faculty/reusch/virttx tjml/special2.htm**

While much of the above reports mean little to most readers, the important thing here is that the chemicals employed are described in layman's terms and are of little apparent consequence.

Therefore, none of the byproducts in any of these reaction sequences are particularly dangerous, nor should they be of any concern in themselves, and none employ high heat. However. Bergstrom Research, as discussed both here elsewhere herein and on their website, selected a distillation method for marketing and their product is specifically marketed to humans. Their claim is that the water used in the several above crystallization sequences compromises the integrity of the MSM sold for animals and that some of the mild chemicals may not be dissipated in these simple and inexpensive sequences.

So Bergstrom settled on a more expensive distillation process that requires more heat, energy, and, considerably more cost, thus allowing them to justify their higher end product cost. They, like many vitamin companies, have no real marketing edge, so they claim a cleaner product. This would be of little consequence if you only took two or three grams as they recommend and employ in their testing. However, the original protocol in my above book suggests as much as ½ cup per day (according to your health condition). In fact, all MSM is fairly free of contamination unless the product sits in storage for long periods. The end argument then, here, is that it is all about quantity and has little to do with quality.

However, as claimed in the above book, the animal MSM (employing crystallization) is the correct product. That is, as related initially by the person who revealed the original protocol, heat may compromise the final product by reducing the bioavailablity of the organic sulfur component of the methylsulfonylmethane. This protocol is not about brands. It does, however, identify animal MSM (the crystallization process) to be the correct form. Furthermore, the sulfur component is thought by most people today, even those quite familiar with MSM, to be the only one active and especially by those unfamiliar with the methylation sequences (which I had little awareness of when I wrote the above book).

I do, however, identify these cellular energy sequences in my second book, "Methylation, Awareness, and You" as most likely one of two pathways were the cure for final stage mesothelioma, a rare form of lung cancer, caused by the ingestion of asbestos in the lungs occurs. These would be as follows:

First, MSM, especially in the very high quantities as described in my books, virtually cleans the body of internal poisons. This first method has been identified by various experts for some thirty years or more in smaller amounts, but higher levels (called HL MSM), apparently magnify these results greatly.

Second, the three methylation pathways, I believe, basically supercharge all three pathways. Today, most experts attribute this to only one of them, but we have plenty of room for study and very little objective, independent study has done. To date, nearly all of the study on MSM for humans has been funded by Bergstrom and, as I point out elsewhere, it is badly flawed and biased to their product. However, it is very likely that the methylation sequences are the key to the above cancer healing, not the organic sulfur.

Cancer, MSM and Vitamin C

So, below, I find a new website devoted to treating cancer with HL MSM:

"The MSM/ Vit C Treatment for Cancer"
http://www.cancertutor.com/faq_msm/
From the website: "The Cancer Tutor"

This report is about 50% correct and it has been compromised by Bergstrom., Bergstrom, again, sells distilled MSM form for people, far inferior to the much cheaper crystallized from my reports. That is, Crystalized MSM as intended for animals as reported elsewhere, herein.

The delivery method of dissolving it in water and drinking it is also a compromise. That is, swishing gets MSM into your system at a much higher rate and, further, it adds saliva which aids in the digestion process for any that finally does reach the stomach (most does not, when

98

swished). Still, until recently, no one knew anything about the HL MSM protocol that I passed to my friends on the web some fifteen years ago and more recently in the book, "It's the Liver Stupid."

This site does not attempt to go into why MSM does what it does for cancer other than its organic sulfur content, which now, with the methylation pathways story, could be concluded to be maybe 1/3 of the story. However, in cancer treatment the sulfur content may actually be none of the story.

The methylation pathways as described in layman's terms in the book "Methylation, Awareness, and You" tell you the 2/3 that was left out. In this case, then, both distilled and crystallized forms,, are likely equal in effect in terms of methylation pathways stimulation. However, still, the crystallized form with its high sulfur delivery levels works best for joint health and that also may augment cancer patients to some degree, since MSM is a great way to remove toxins.

Finally, if you are diagnosed with cancer, you should be taking at least ½ cup per day in divided doses and maybe more. Why not? You need all of the help that you can get and now we know that it does provide powerful immunity help in many ways. Certainly, MSM is probably the best "system vacuum cleaner" in the world. Especially, if you believe that toxins do cause cancer as this website concludes, you would be well advised to get them out of your system quickly. In fact, most experts today agree with the idea that toxins do set up the grounds for cancer and removing the cause can create a cure.

Age Erasing

Dr. David Struthers' book "Age Erasing" **http://nickpineault.org/age-eraser-review-is-age-eraser-net-scam-or-legit** is a controversial book on removing the effects of aging as it well should be. His methods, while generally good advice do not affect the microcellular events that cause and keep aging. Certainly, advising people to remove nervous tension from their lives would be helpful in antiaging if anyone could achieve that. However, no one consciously creates tension, so if they knew how, they would reduce it consciously and they cause it unconsciously of course. There are spiritual tricks that can be learned and practiced that have these effects, but a person must be ready to do them and most are not or they would be now.

As to his supplement advice:

Struthers never mentions Vitamin D3 and adequate sunlight as antiaging. In fact, he still parrots the old advice to avoid sunlight entirely. Chances are that he would add that we must use adequate sun block, etc. Face it, you only normally get one antiquated course in nutrition in med school, so how would this prepare you for being the antiaging advisor that he claims to be?

Facial Creams

He recommends facial creams etc., but seems to rely on commercial preparations. The fact is that most commercial preparations make you feel good about your skin, but the long term effect is nil. Probably the most effective skin treatment in the world is to spray ocean water on your body daily followed by the skin cream that you prepare as offered in formula in the "It's the Liver Stupid." This is all very simple, cheap to do, and fast. You do this after a hot shower when the skin pores are wide open.

Astaxanthan

This is still the most likely product available on the market to help in removing the aging characteristics of skin. This is the orange pigment that gives lobsters, crayfish, and flamingos their protective orange pigment. For those of us who respect the wisdom of nature, this is what nature produces as a protection against getting too much sun, not sun lotion. Yes, while not getting enough sun is an aging factor, too much is also. But the mainstream is far less than 50% correct in their warnings.

However, you will find that if you take astaxanthin on a daily basis and use it in a skin preparation, you will never sunburn again even if you, by mistake, get too much sun. This the author has proven to himself. However, do not take this as a recommendation to experiment in this area. About 15 minutes of direct full sun over the entire body per day is apparently adequate to fill our D3 needs without supplementation. This, of course, has everything to do with skin pigmentation, which determine your rate of absorbency, so you must adjust it to more when your complection is darker. One might think of themselves as a solar panel and D3 as the storage unit in this equation. Obviously, our bodies are much more complex, but the analysis is still pretty good.

In Closing:

So I have walked you through the most profound results of the new quantum science that is just revealing itself everyday with leaps and bounds. This, as my friend, Dr. Rich Price works with people all over the world and, in many cases, heals them of previously untreatable diseases and often in just hours.

At the same time, I have advanced the basis for why the HL MSM works to some degree, herein, and given some of the advancements reported over the past five years of those who have ventured into this simple protocol that always worked for osteoarthritis, joint and muscle pain, but is now showing promise for allergies, asthma, and even cancer.

The point here is that when we do the work and pay attention, we can be well and live far longer than any of our recent ancestors and maintain a high level of health at virtually any age.

Update on Dr. Price's Work:

The newest work, that may be the most important yet, that Dr. Richard Price has done is to effect a resistance (cure if you will) to harmful frequency fields as they effect the human body and especially Electromagnetic (EM) as follows:

Read first Wiki's comprehesive definition of all forms of invisble and visible radiation frequencies at:
https://en.wikipedia.org/wiki/Electromagnetic_spectru m
Most of our aware population realize the significant problems that EM causes to the the human body when so exposed and we must realize that our bodies were not designed to fight off EM frequencies. Just as all scientists agree that the effects of a nuclear blast and its resulting nuclear activity as well as X-rays from medical testing will quickly cause cellular damage so will EM. These changes can easily cause cancer and are basically poisons to our systems. In fact, Rich's treatment will also make your body resistant to all forms of foreign radiation.

Next, read here how the Van Allen Belt protects us at: **https://en.wikipedia.org/wiki/Van_Allen_radiation_belt**)

While the Belt is discussed as causing problems with NASA missions, Seldom do we hear of just how an intercontinental flight can cause EM problems for people or standing in front of a microwave oven not well shielded can. Or, as Dan Nelson discusses, how EM can alter water that is heated or that it can remove all nutrients from food.

Today, we also have the thermonuclear reactor meltdown in Fukishima to add more concerns as the west to east weather carries radiation to the east coast of the US at rising levels. Some scientists claim that we have about two years left before the levels become unsustainable.

The positive long-term affects of this work can easily surpass any single disease treatment so far and as time goes on, they will become more important I predict.

Growing Young Gracefully

>I apply coconut oil on my skin in the sauna is that okay?<

In answering you, I describe the basic processes behind growing young and, indeed, point to how that occurs. Your sauna question is, no doubt an attempt at this, but it is a small subset of many processes that must occur to make it all happen. So read on please and keep an open mind:

The first fact is that the skin is a better place to get nutrients than orally (except as I iterate below). If you want coconut oil in your body, apply it externally and you will get it. And, yes, open pores help a lot. So, after a shower or in a sauna you enhance the process as heat opens the pores. The pores of the skin move nutrients through them much more quickly than anyone imagines. Read my references to Dr. Mark Sircus below and elsewhere for his very well studied information on this topic.

I would not overdo coconut oil, but it is a fine nutrient compared to most things that people eat and call foods as it is seldom or never tainted with chemicals. One thing that you might consider is sea salt sprayed on your skin. My first book, "It's the Liver Stupid" has a formula for a mixture of many nutrients that include astaxanthin which is a powerful skin protectant as well as one of the most powerful antioxidants in the world.

If you watch Dr. Dan Nelson's Water video, **https://www.google.com/#q=Dan+Nelson+water** he mentions going into a grocery store and measuring the health contents of all products and basically getting nothing. I can affirm what he measured as I have affirmed his results. Only the produce isle has a chance at real health as he states and often those products are grown

105

under terrible conditions. Fat is very good for you as it is concentrated food and you do not need much, but this is where our cattle and poultry store the toxins that they are raised on. You will notice that cats and dogs always eat fat first as it is the highest energy source normally, but in today's world, it is not the most healthy... and meats generally are the opposite of what our ancestors sought out as the most valuable food source that they once were. Sea food sounds good. But you must ask, Was it caught off the shores of the Fukishima Reactors? Green foods generally are awesome when from good sources, but they are not good energy sources and they are hard to digest comparative.

The point above is that it is harder and harder to make good choices as our food is manufactured and mass produced, but coconuts are generally a good bet to be clean and pure and coconut oil is very healthful as a dietary element. But we need variety and that is the root of our problem here.

Transdermal has the added benefit of not having to go through the digestive process which costs the body about 90% of what it makes (as I measure it). Caloric count, which the mainstream relies on so heavily, we have found, is only a small piece of the dietary puzzle. If it were as important as we are led to believe, would our population be so overweight? However, mainstream science as you will see at
http://community.myfitnesspal.com/en/discussion/4821

81/how-efficient-is-the-human-digestive-system still sees protein, carbohydrates and calories as the whole picture and thus our misleading food pyramid as published by the FDA. You could conceivably get all of your nutrients transdermally and that would be 100% efficient, but in doing that, you would avoid the body's natural internal digestive defense systems, so you had better be making the correct choices in doing this or you could poison yourself in short order. I doubt anyone has tried this, but who knows? Dr. Mark Sircus is the transdermal guru **http://drsircus.com/about-dr-sircus-treatment-method** of our times and he is a great source of information on this topic that you have raised.

My own interest is in anti-aging medicine (if it really is a medicine... I see it as far more than that today as I learn). To see where the mainstream is with this "specialty," read **http://www.a4m.com/conferences-attendees-what-is-anti-aging-medicine.html**. The truth is that these mainstream Newtonians have no idea where to start in this most exciting area. The thing that got me here was my MSM discovery and its implications that are slowly being revealed by the readers of my first book. I guessed right in many places there and, yes, I was somewhat lucky, but high levels of MSM certainly reduce aging factors at a rate far greater than any of these mainstream data points, but there is more.

We have known for many years now that our Newtonian, now Genetic based, biology has it wrong and the real

107

science is occurring at the quantum level... the microcellular level and with that, the sub-conscious and spiritual level. My first book started out here, but again, I was lucky. At this point, I consider it as excellent inner guidance and not luck, but the fact is that quantum biology can make you well and keep you there. As the brilliant Bruce Lipton, below, tells you, genes are just blue prints and they are otherwise inactive. If blue prints did work, I could project mine at a jobsite and produce buildings. It is too bad that I cannot as that would save a great deal of work, but they are still helpful in making buildings happen.

What common anti-aging supplements work? The answer is, most likely, none. However, they return more cash than cocaine does to the doctors who sell them and many, like synthetic HGH, can be deadly. Most supplements hawked by the mainstream are poisons just as are cosmetics. Mainstream mufti-vitamins are poisons. FDA approval means that no one could prove that it will harm you in the short term. We are discussing long term here. Weight control based on dietary restrictions and long periods of exercise do almost nothing in making you younger.

We have been and are being lied to by the mainstream press. This is not likely to change anytime soon and this all comes down to politics, not health. Even those who write against anti-aging seldom have any idea what the root problems are, but there will never be any helpful solutions to this from the Newtonian Mainstream biology and science on either side. It simply cannot happen. It is like searching your house car keys that are stuck in the ignition switch. Quantum Science, once you understand it, is not even measurable using Newtonian devised instruments so how would they know anything? This is a new game.

The bottom line is that single most important anti-aging factor is between your ears (but this is not even totally accurate because mind does not occur there. It occurs around and outside there).

This is just the beginning of what we have discovered, but even the mainstream tells you that anti-aging medicine can increase lifespan by 20 to 800% with facts and figures. However , the real fact is that when done well, 800% is a just a spit in the ocean, but it will take several hundred years to prove. So the greatest single attribute to anti-aging is reduced stress levels and the 2nd is diet. Mainstream doctors have no idea what the correct diet should be. Also, they can't alter microcellular health where it all starts.

Watch
https://www.youtube.com/watch?v=zwOvg1rJfcM Dr. Bruce Lipton has a powerful understanding of how energy works within the cells at these ultra small quantum levels where our interest should be concentrated. You really should listen to all of his You Tube lectures if you are interested in staying young and well.

At some point, Bruce tells you that age is just a number that you have bought into. Sure, it has meaning in that it measures where you have been. But your interest should be in where you are going and what your attitude is in going there. Once you understand the real factors involved in aging, suddenly, this becomes the first day of your life and you control where it is going, not drugs or genes.

Edocrene disruptors

https://www.youtube.com/watch?v=PunH8kdjhJw

This is probably the most comprehensive overview of the most critical health issues today available.

You must know a little about everything everything that this doctor has to report if you ever plan to be a healthy person today. At some point, I have hit fairly hard on every point that he makes here in this or one of my previous books. He goes over about everyone in some detail, but not great depth. For instance, one need not be an expert on asbestos to know that brake dust can cause serious health issues. Just about every aspect of our lives today can contribute serious issues when it comes to the endocrene system if we do not avoid them as much as possible.

We are not going to avoid hormone disruptors entirely, but HL MSM does help eliminate them due to the methyl and sulfur components and in many cases very quickly, as readers report So without huge changes in our environment, we can never avoid even a small percentage of these toxins and MSM can help ameliorate them as others report.

GcMAF, Miracle Cure?

There is a good deal of talk about this relatively newly discovered natural drug.

"So what is GcMAF? It's a protein that is normally found in the blood of healthy people. It is an immunomodulatory protein, in that its activity affects the function of the immune system. The glycoprotein (a protein with sugar molecules attached) GcMAF results from sequential deglycosylation of the vitamin D-binding protein (the Gc protein), and the resulting protein is felt to be a macrophage activating factor (MAF)."

"MAFs are a class of protein known as a lymphokine, and they regulate the expression of antigens on the surface of macrophages. One of their functions is to "activate" macrophages, which can under the proper circumstances attack cancer cells. Of note, the production of GcMAF can be blocked by an enzyme called Nagalase (alpha-N-acetylgalactosaminidase), produced by many cancers, which led to its first incarnation in quackery as a "cure" for many cancers by Bill Sardi and Timothy Hubbell, based on dubious science and a clinical trial that didn't

show what its proponents claimed it did and was later
retracted."
https://www.sciencebasedmedicine.org/gcmaf-and-the-l

Made in the USA
Middletown, DE
14 April 2020